Reproductive Medicine for the MRCOG

Reproductive Medicine for the MRCOG

Edited by

Siladitya Bhattacharya
University of Aberdeen

Mark Hamilton
University of Aberdeen

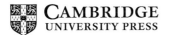

CAMBRIDGE
UNIVERSITY PRESS

University Printing House, Cambridge CB2 8BS, United Kingdom

One Liberty Plaza, 20th Floor, New York, NY 10006, USA

477 Williamstown Road, Port Melbourne, VIC 3207, Australia

314–321, 3rd Floor, Plot 3, Splendor Forum, Jasola District Centre, New Delhi – 110025, India

79 Anson Road, #06–04/06, Singapore 079906

Cambridge University Press is part of the University of Cambridge.

It furthers the University's mission by disseminating knowledge in the pursuit of
education, learning, and research at the highest international levels of excellence.

www.cambridge.org
Information on this title: www.cambridge.org/9781108817837
DOI: 10.1017/9781108861724

© Siladitya Bhattacharya and Mark Hamilton 2021

First published 2021

Printed in the United Kingdom by TJ Books Limited, Padstow Cornwall

A catalogue record for this publication is available from the British Library.

ISBN 978-1-108-81783-7 Paperback

Contents

Contributors

Richard A. Anderson, MD, PhD, FRCOG
MRC Centre for Reproductive Health, University of Edinburgh, and Edinburgh Fertility and Reproductive Endocrinology Centre, Royal Infirmary, Edinburgh, Scotland

Sarah Armstrong, MBChB, MRCOG
The University of Sheffield, Department of Oncology and Metabolism, Medical School, Sheffield, England

Siladitya Bhattacharya, MD, FRCOG
Head of School of Medicine, Medical Sciences and Nutrition and Clinical Chair of Obstetrics and Gynaecology, University of Aberdeen, Foresterhill, Aberdeen; Honorary Consultant NHS Grampian, Aberdeen Fertility Centre, Aberdeen Maternity Hospital, Aberdeen, Scotland

Virginia N. Bolton, MA, PhD
Former Consultant Clinical Embryologist, Guy's Assisted Conception Unit, Guy's Hospital, London, UK

Jacky Boivin, B.A., M.A., PhD, CPsychol
School of Psychology (Cardiff Fertility Studies Research Group), College of Biomedical and Life Sciences, Cardiff University, Cardiff, Wales

Maya Chetty, MD, MRCOG
Edinburgh Fertility and Reproductive Endocrinology Centre, Royal Infirmary, Edinburgh, Scotland

Cynthia Farquhar, CNZM, FRSNZ, MBChB, FRCOG, FRANZCOG, CREI, MPH, MD
Postgraduate Professor of Obstetrics and Gynaecology, Department of Obstetrics and Gynaecology, Faculty of Medical and Health Sciences, School of Medicine, University of Auckland, Auckland, New Zealand; Coordinating Editor, Cochrane Gynaecology and Fertility; Senior Editor,

Cochrane Abdomen and Endocrine Network; Clinical Director of Gynaecology, National Women's Health + Auckland District Health Board, Auckland, New Zealand

Mark Hamilton, MD, FRCOG
Honorary Clinical Senior Lecturer, University of Aberdeen, Aberdeen Maternity Hospital Foresterhill, Aberdeen, Scotland

Haitham Hamoda, MD, FRCOG
King's College Hospital NHS Foundation Trust, London, England

Gillian Lockwood, FRCOG, DPhil, MA (Oxon)
Medical Director, CARE Fertility Tamworth, Tamworth, England

Abha Maheshwari, MBBS, MD, FRCOG
Consultant in Reproductive Medicine & Surgery, Aberdeen Fertility Centre, Aberdeen Maternity Hospital, Aberdeen, Scotland

Kevin McEleny, BSc (Hons), PhD, FRCS (Urol)
Consultant Urologist, Newcastle Fertility Centre, The Newcastle-upon-Tyne Hospitals NHS Trust, International Centre For Life, Newcastle-upon-Tyne, England

Alison McTavish, RGN, RM
Business & Quality Manager, Aberdeen Centre for Reproductive Medicine, Aberdeen, Scotland

Ben Willem Mol, FRANZCOG, PhD
Department of Obstetrics and Gynaecology, Monash Health, VIC, Australia

Andrew William Nguyen, BBiomedSc, BMedSc (Hons), MD
Faculty of Medicine, Nursing and Health Sciences, Monash University, VIC, Australia

Petra Nordqvist, BSc, MSc, MSc, PhD
Senior Lecturer, Department of Sociology (Morgan Centre for Research in Everyday Lives), School of Social Sciences, The University of Manchester, Manchester, England

Allan Pacey, MBE, PhD, FRCOG
Professor of Andrology, Department of Oncology and Metabolism, University of Sheffield, Sheffield, South Yorkshire, England

Lucky Saraswat, MBBS, MRCOG, PhD
Consultant Gynaecologist, Aberdeen Royal Infirmary; Honorary Senior Lecturer, University of Aberdeen, Aberdeen, Scotland

Sesh K. Sunkara, MBBS, MD, FRCOG
Department of Women's Health, King's College London, England

Petra Thorn, DGSF
Social worker, social and family therapist, private practice, Möorfelden, Germany

Kugajeevan Vigneswaran, MBBS, MRCOG
King's College Hospital NHS Foundation Trust, London, England

Epidemiology and Initial Assessment of the Infertile Patient

Mark Hamilton

1.1 Introduction

This chapter discusses the epidemiology of infertility and the importance of the initial assessment of people with infertility. Profound changes in society over the past two decades challenge previously agreed upon norms in our understanding of the nature of parenthood and family. Defining infertility in a contemporary context has thus also changed as the profile of those seeking advice has evolved. Nevertheless, it remains essential that efficient mechanisms for referral and investigation are established for those involved in the planning of fertility services. These must involve a good liaison between primary care providers and medical, nursing and diagnostic laboratory staff in specialist centres. Adherence to agreed upon protocols will facilitate appropriate and timely investigation along standardised paths, thereby minimising risk of delay and repetition of tests which those seeking assistance find particularly demoralising. Once a diagnosis is reached it should be possible to offer people with infertility an accurate prognosis and the opportunity to consider the issues relevant to treatment choices for their particular situation.

1.2 Epidemiology

The International Glossary on Infertility and Fertility Care (2017) [1] highlighted the importance of rigour in using terms and definitions relevant to fertility care. It is now acknowledged that infertility is a disease of the reproductive system which in some instances leads to significant disability. Acceptance of this has, in many countries, been a major driver in establishing equity of access to care, though in the United Kingdom this remains an as yet unmet challenge.

Fecundity is a term describing the natural capacity of a woman to have a live birth. Fecundability refers to the chance of a pregnancy being established during a single menstrual cycle, in a woman with adequate exposure to sperm and who is not using contraception, which leads to a live birth. In population studies fecundability is usually measured as a monthly probability.

The Total Fertility Rate (TFR) refers to the average number of live births a woman will have in the totality of her reproductive life. This may be determined in retrospect to an individual through observed data. If applied to a group of women, for example, all women in a certain year, it is referred to as a Cohort Total Fertility Rate (CTFR) and is determined after all women have completed their reproductive years. In England and Wales the TFR in 2017 was 1.76 births per woman. This represented the fifth year in succession in which the rate had declined. In 2012 the level was 1.94 (Figure 1.1).

The Age-Specific Fertility Rate (ASFR) describes the number of live births per woman in a particular age group in a specific calendar year expressed per 1,000 women in that age group. This has declined in every age group in recent years except for women older than 40 years, in whom there has been an increase, with levels now at their highest since 1949. Delaying childbirth and the impact of fertility treatments in older women are major influences on these interesting trends.

The TFR can also be estimated for a population of women over a defined period of time. The Period Total Fertility Rate (PTFR) is the number of children who would be born per woman (or per 1,000 women) if she/they were to pass through the childbearing years bearing children according to a current schedule of age-specific fertility rates. The figure is obtained by adding up the single-year ASFRs over the defined period.

Another concept which bears consideration is that of the TFR level required to sustain population levels in particular countries. This 'replacement fertility rate' in the developed world is of the order of 2.1, though in developing countries the figure may be much higher due to increased mortality rates, particularly among children.

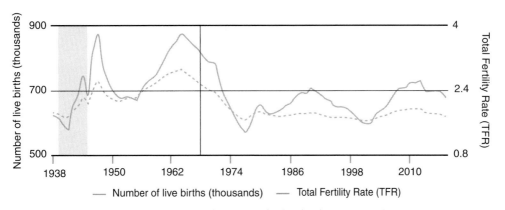

Figure 1.1 Number of live births and Total Fertility Rate (England and Wales) (1938–2017).

Data accessed from Office for National Statistics (UK)

www.ons.gov.uk/peoplepopulationandcommunity/birthsdeathsandmarriages/livebirths/bulletins/birthsummarytablesenglandandwales/2017

Analysis of global population trends shows a decline in TFR in many developed countries. In the United Kingdom in 2017 the rate was 1.7 whereas in 1950 this figure was 4.7. In sub-Saharan Africa the figures for TFR are higher, for example, Uganda 5.2. In many other areas of the world the TFR is very low and much below that required to sustain population levels. Three key factors are involved in these trends – fewer deaths in childhood mean women today have fewer babies; men and women have greater access to contraception; and more women are in education and working. Age at first birth is rising in many countries and in the United Kingdom is now approaching 30 years. Among women born in 1972 the average age at first birth is 31 years. For women born in 1945 the figure was 23–24 years. The consequence of these trends will have a significant effect on the demography of populations, with fewer young people available to resource the care of an increasingly aged population. Migration may to a degree mitigate against these trends but the problems for some countries will have very profound implications for society in the future.

In any population, not all women without children at the end of their reproductive life are infertile. Voluntary childlessness is not an uncommon lifestyle choice. Involuntary childlessness, however, may be a consequence of not establishing a life partnership with a member of the opposite sex, or where a person has had the misfortune of all children having died. A major cause of involuntary childlessness, however, is infertility. Same-sex relationships are an established societal norm in many parts of the world and thus infertility as a term now has to take account of the potential use of third-party reproductive techniques in assisting those seeking to have a child and where, after exposure to treatment over a defined period of time, pregnancy has failed to establish and no live birth has ensued.

In practice the term 'infertility' can be interchangeable with 'subfertility' although it is debatable as to whether the term subfertility is useful. Sterility should be regarded as a permanent state of infertility. The Glossary defines infertility as 'a disease characterised by the failure to establish a clinical pregnancy after 12 months of regular unprotected intercourse, or due to impairment in a person's capacity to reproduce either as an individual or with his/her partner'.

The use of the specific time frame is both necessary and based on sound epidemiological data. The length of exposure time considered is determined by the observation that in the general population, which would include a proportion of couples with infertility, one would expect the chance of a woman becoming pregnant in any individual cycle (fecundability) to be around 20%. By 1 year of exposure about 85% of couples would have established a pregnancy and by the time 2 years has elapsed this figure will have reached 92% [2]. For couples presenting with more than 4 years' unwanted childlessness the prospects for becoming pregnant without assistance are very low. In practical terms the failure to achieve pregnancy causes enormous distress to those affected. For people with fertility problems, using a definition of a year to describe infertility is usual and most will have sought medical advice or assistance by that time.

Age-specific fertility rates for women decline in association with increasing age, though in an ultimately fertile group of women it is not certain that their monthly fecundability (% chance of establishing a pregnancy leading to a live birth) is any less than in younger cohorts. It may be sensible to consider specialist referral of women over the age of 35 years in advance of 1 year. However, it should be recognised that in many instances pregnancy will be established without medical assistance in these cases, since it can be assumed that a proportion will not be infertile.

Infertility is often categorised as either primary or secondary. Primary female infertility refers to a woman who has never been diagnosed with a clinical pregnancy. Primary male infertility refers to a man who has never initiated a clinical pregnancy. In both instances women and men should meet the criteria for the definition of infertility. Secondary female infertility refers to a woman unable to establish a clinical pregnancy who has previously been diagnosed with a clinical pregnancy. Secondary male infertility refers to a man who has previously initiated a clinical pregnancy but is now unable to do so. A clinical pregnancy refers to a pregnancy diagnosed by ultrasonographic visualisation of one or more gestation sacs within the uterus or definitive clinical signs of pregnancy or a clinically documented ectopic pregnancy.

Estimates of the prevalence of infertility in the population are influenced by the duration of infertility used in the definition and the setting of the population studied, for example, primary care or hospital clinics. Community-based data will give the most accurate reflection of prevalence within the general population but these studies are few in number. Published prevalence studies suggest a range of lifetime risk of infertility varying from 6.6% to 32.6%. One population-based study in the north east of Scotland which took account also of pregnancies resulting in miscarriage and ectopic pregnancy found a prevalence of 14% using a 2-year definition.

In global terms the prevalence of infertility seems to have changed little in the last 20 years. In the United Kingdom setting a number of factors have been a matter of concern with respect to their potential impact on the prevalence of infertility. These include the incidence of sexually transmitted infection (STI) such as *Chlamydia trachomatis* in the young. In addition, there have been suggestions that environmental factors may affect male fertility. As alluded to earlier, profound questions have been raised about the effects on female fertility of delayed childbearing as determined by changes in lifestyle and working patterns. Despite these legitimate concerns, when the population-based study was repeated [3] the observed prevalence of infertility had not increased in north east Scotland in the succeeding 20 years.

Data from a review of worldwide prevalence studies, using a 5-year definition and live birth as the outcome, suggest that nearly 50 million couples worldwide are infertile. This includes 1.9% of couples wishing to have a first child who have primary infertility and 10.5% of those who have previously had a live birth experiencing secondary infertility. Regional variations were noted in this study in the overall prevalence, particularly in relation to secondary infertility with, in some Eastern European; South-East Asian; and West, Central and Southern African countries, more than 20% of couples affected (Figure 1.2). This is most likely due to the prevalence of infective complications following miscarriage, abortion or childbirth as well as the acquisition of sexually transmitted infections in these settings. A previous study using a shorter duration of infertility as the definition suggested the worldwide figure could be as high as 80 million couples. This review also suggested that the overall prevalence of infertility changed very little worldwide between 1990 and 2010.

A lack of observed change in prevalence should not encourage complacency in respect of public health responsibilities. Opportunities to prevent infertility are limited, and encouragement to the young to engage in safe sexual practices limiting exposure to risk of STI is clearly important. For teenage girls, rubella immunisation programmes should be in place. HPV vaccination programmes are now established. Education of the public about the known decline in fertility which occurs with age, particularly in women older than 35 years of age, is also important. Furthermore, the need for folic acid supplementation for women to reduce the risk of neural tube defect should be promoted as well as the need to make certain lifestyle adjustments on issues such as the potential need to moderate levels of smoking and alcohol consumption as well as achieving optimal weight. There is convincing evidence that smoking, active or passive, affects reproductive performance in women, and men, as well as increasing the risks in pregnancy of small for gestational age infants,

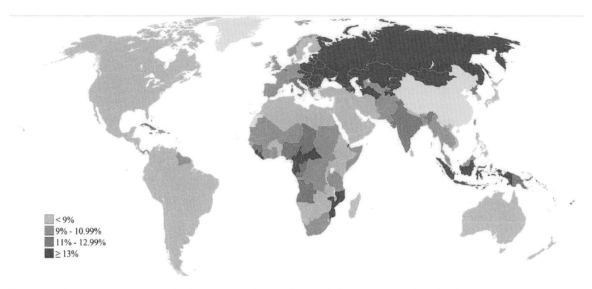

Figure 1.2 Prevalence of secondary infertility among women who have had a live birth previously and seek another, in 2010.
Data from: Mascarenhas MN, Flaxman SR, Boerma T, Vanderpoel S, Stevens GA.
National, Regional, and Global Trends in Infertility Prevalence since 1990:
A Systematic Analysis of 277 Health Surveys.
PLoS Med 2012;9(12): e1001356.

stillbirth and infant mortality. Referral to a smoking cessation programme to support efforts in stopping smoking should be available to those who find giving up the habit difficult. Chronic high stress may also have deleterious effects on the biology of reproduction in both men and women as well as have an impact on sexual frequency and performance.

Our public health responsibilities as reproductive medicine specialists thus lie not just in providing fertility care but also in providing people with information and support in planning families and avoiding pregnancy where wished. We also have a professional responsibility to ensure that women are provided with safe services in relation to unwanted pregnancy and miscarriage as well as safe care in pregnancy and childbirth.

1.3 Initial Assessment

1.3.1 Primary Care

In our UK setting the role of the general practitioner is crucial. Infertility represents a deeply personal problem, and many individuals will prefer to discuss intimate matters with someone they know and trust. The support that the GP can provide in terms of counselling and preliminary investigations is an excellent foundation for provision of care. Not infrequently the man and woman may be registered with different GPs. One should always consider that infertility is a problem affecting both parties and each may contribute to the pathogenesis. Once referral is made to a specialist clinic the stresses imposed on couples may increase, with demands on their time for attendance, the indignity of some of the investigations carried out and the invasion of privacy that occurs. Since it is well recognised that infertility investigation and treatment pose real threats to domestic stability, it is the GP, through knowledge of the couple and their families, who may be in the best position to provide support for those struggling to come to terms with continued disappointment.

All patients should be seen as couples in appropriate surroundings. Facilities should be available to permit examination of both partners and with sufficient time, usually half an hour, set aside to make an adequate overall assessment of the problem.

It may be helpful for the local fertility clinic to employ dedicated liaison staff to assist with the referral process and guideline dissemination. In some instances, tubal assessment might be organised in primary care, though before committing to intrusive investigation it would be wise to have information on semen quality beforehand. This can be difficult where the male partner has a different GP than the female partner, but improved communication within primary care can resolve this issue. Bearing in mind the statutory requirement in offering licensed treatment to take account of the welfare of the potential child or existing children it is essential that GPs give this some thought at this early stage to avoid difficulties in later management.

1.3.2 Specialist Centre Care

This should be provided in a setting under the clinical direction of a consultant gynaecologist with a special interest in infertility. Patients should be seen in a dedicated infertility clinic with appropriate appointment times to permit thorough evaluation. A team system should be established involving medical, nursing, laboratory (endocrine and andrology) and counselling personnel to facilitate a consistent and co-ordinated approach to care. The level of treatment options available will depend on the expertise of, and the facilities available to, staff at each centre.

1.3.3 The Infertility Consultation

The point at which any couple might seek assistance will be influenced by a number of factors, not least the degree of anxiety which couples feel in confronting seemingly relentless monthly disappointments. Any couple worried about their fertility should thus be seen by their GP, regardless of the duration of their infertility. It is unusual for couples to present if this is less than a year but it may be apparent to individuals that they may be at risk of a fertility problem and seek advice at an early stage. For example, the man may have had a vasectomy, or undergone testicular surgery in childhood, for example, orchidopexy; either partner may be a survivor of childhood cancer and have undergone chemotherapy; or the woman may be aware of an association of absent or irregular periods with infertility. For some a concern through the high profile which infertility now attracts in the media may have eroded self-assurance about personal fecundity. Unless there is a clear need on the basis of history or examination of either partner, further investigation is usually unnecessary, if the duration of infertility is less than 1 year. Providing the couple with an outline of their excellent fertility potential may be all that is required to set their minds at rest. However, couples

who present early may themselves have particular concerns or have problems which merit sympathetic discussion. A little more urgency may also be required in the investigation of couples where the female partner is over 35 years of age.

Three simple questions require to be addressed in the assessment of infertile individuals:

1. Are sperm available?
That is, is there evidence of normal sperm production and ejaculatory competence?

2. Are eggs available?
That is, is the woman ovulating?

3. Can the gametes meet?
That is, is female pelvic anatomy normal and is coital function adequate?

Steps in the process of investigation of infertility should be discussed at the outset with the couple in the expectation that all necessary tests would be complete within 4 months. The sequence with which tests are performed is, to some extent, standardised for all but may vary if history or examination findings suggest otherwise. Initial investigations are inexpensive, non-invasive and likely to yield useful information.

Points requiring particular attention in the history and examination of the couple are shown in Tables 1.1 and 1.2.

A psychological assessment of the impact of perceived infertility on individuals and the couple is an essential component of this initial encounter. Libido and consequently coital frequency may be profoundly influenced by the experience of infertility and thus affect prognosis.

1.4 Preliminary Investigations

1.4.1 Male

Semen analysis remains the most important means of assessment. It is desirable, in order to avoid unhelpful and frustrating duplication, for GP-referred assessments to take place in the same laboratory which serves the clinic to which the couple may ultimately be referred. Clear instructions on the provision of samples should be given: a period of abstinence of at least 3 days but no longer than 1 week is desirable; the sample should be kept at body temperature in transportation and should arrive at the laboratory if being provided off site within 1 hour of production. In most instances a single sample will suffice if the result is normal. If

Table 1.1 Initial assessment of female infertility: history and examination

Area of investigation	History	Area of investigation	Examination
Infertility	Duration of infertility Length and type of contraceptive use Fertility in previous relationships as well as in present liaison Previous investigation and treatment Fertility subsequently, if known, in any former partners Previous fertility investigations and treatment	General	Height, weight, BMI Fat and hair distribution (Ferriman–Gallwey score to quantify hirsutism) Note presence or absence of acne and galactorrhoea.
Medical	Menstrual history: • Menarche • Cycle length and duration of flow • Pain • Bouts of amenorrhoea • Menorrhagia • Intermenstrual bleeding Number of previous pregnancies including abortions, miscarriages and ectopic pregnancies Any associated sepsis Time to initiate previous pregnancies Drug history past and present: for example, agents which cause hyperprolactinaemia, past cytotoxic treatment or radiotherapy	Abdominal	Check for abdominal masses or tenderness.
Surgical	Previous abdominal or pelvic surgery in particular gynaecological procedures	Pelvis	Assess state of hymen. Assess normality of clitoris and labia. Assess vagina, looking for such problems as infection or vaginal septa, endometriotic deposits. Check for presence of cervical polyps. Assess accessibility of the cervix for insemination. Record uterine size, position, mobility and tenderness. Perform cervical smear if appropriate.
Occupational	Work patterns including separation from partner		
Sexual	Coital frequency and timing, including knowledge of the fertile period Dyspareunia Post-coital bleeding		

an abnormality is found then the sample should be repeated, usually after 1 month, though resolution of any transient insult leading to defects in sperm production may not be apparent for up to 3 months. If a gross abnormality is noted, for example, azoospermia, the sample may be repeated within a short time interval.

What constitutes a normal result is a matter of debate. Large laboratories may have their own local population based normal ranges, but in the absence of local information the World Health Organization values for definition of normality can be applied [5] (Table 1.3). Such definitions of normality as predictors of pregnancy are poor. More complex tests of sperm function, including their potential for movement, cervical mucus penetration, capacitation, zona recognition, the acrosome reaction and sperm–oocyte fusion, have been developed but in practice are rarely required. Further detailed discussion of the assessment and treatment of male factor infertility is given in Chapter 5.

Table 1.2 Initial assessment of male infertility: history and examination

Area of investigation	History	Area of investigation	Examination
Infertility	Duration of infertility Fertility in previous relationships as well as in present liaison Fertility subsequently, if known, in any former partners Previous fertility investigations and treatment	General	Height, weight, BMI Fat and hair distribution Evidence of hypoandrogenism or gynaecomastia
Medical	Sexually transmitted infection Epididymitis Mumps orchitis Testicular maldescent Chronic disease Drug/alcohol abuse Recent febrile illness Recurrent urinary tract infection	Groin	Exclude inguinal hernia (patient in upright position) Check for inguinal mass e.g. ectopic testicle
Surgical	Herniorrhaphy Testicular injury Torsion Orchidopexy Vasectomy and/or reversal	Genitalia	Note site of testicles in the scrotum an measure volume using an orchidometer Palpate epididymis for nodularity or tenderness Check presence and normality of the vasa deferentia Check for the presence of a varicocele Examine penis for any structural abnormality e.g. hypospadias
Occupational	Toxic substance exposure including chemicals, radiation Time away from home through work		
Sexual	Onset of puberty Coital habits Premature ejaculation Libido/impotence Use and knowledge of the fertile period		

Table 1.3 Laboratory reference range for semen characteristics

Semen parameter	Lower reference limit (5th centiles + 95% confidence intervals)
Semen volume (mL)	1.5 (1.4–1.7)
Total sperm number ($\times 10^6$ per ejaculate)	39 (33–46)
Sperm concentration ($\times 10^6$ per mL)	15 (12–16)
Total motility: progressive + non-progressive (%)	40 (38–42)
Progressive motility (%)	32 (31–34)
Sperm morphology (normal forms, %)	4 (3.0–4.0)

From WHO (2010).

1.4.2 Female

At the outset it is advisable to ensure that the woman has received rubella immunisation, and that she is taking folic acid (0.4 mg/day) to reduce the chance of the fetus developing a neural tube defect (NTD). There may be particular circumstances where a higher dose of folic acid (5 mg) is recommended, for example, patients taking anti-epileptic medication, obese individuals (BMI >30 kg/m^2), either partner or previous child with NTD, or women with diabetes, coeliac disease or thalassaemia. It is recommended that folic acid supplementation continue up to 12 weeks of gestation.

The preliminary investigation centres on the need to demonstrate that the woman is ovulating. This is almost certainly the case if she has a regular monthly cycle. Laboratory evidence may be obtained through measurement of serum progesterone in the putative luteal phase of the menstrual cycle. Levels would be expected to be in excess of 30 nmol/L 7 days after ovulation but levels lower than this do not necessarily preclude the chance that ovulation is occurring. For this reason, sampling should be arranged for day 21 in the context of a 28-day cycle, with serial checks made beyond this point if the cycle is more prolonged or variable in length. Results should be interpreted only in relation to the onset of the subsequent period. If the level is below 20 nmol/L the test may be repeated in a subsequent cycle. In the absence of any clues in history or examination to suggest the possibility of an endocrine disorder these tests would be sufficient. If, however, there is a history of irregular menstruation, or periods of amenorrhoea, in particular if associated with galactorrhoea, hirsutism or obesity, then additional biochemical tests are appropriate. This might include measures of thyroid function, prolactin and androgen production. This will be discussed further in Chapter 2. Robust evidence to suggest that the use of temperature charts and luteinising hormone (LH) detection methods to time intercourse increases the chance of conception is lacking and their routine use should be discouraged.

Thyroid function screening is now routinely offered to all women with infertility. Subclinical hypothyroidism is thought to be associated with an increased risk of miscarriage. It is recommended that serum thyroid-stimulating hormone (TSH) levels should be <2.5 mU/L in women pre-pregnancy in order to prevent early pregnancy loss and optimise obstetric and perinatal outcomes. If levels are higher than this, then screening for thyroid autoantibodies should be carried out. If antibody testing is positive, then low-dose thyroxine replacement therapy (25–50 µg/day) should be initiated to achieve a serum TSH <2.5 mU/L. If autoantibody screening is negative, then it is suggested that repeat testing of TSH should be carried out in 6 months. If the serum TSH level is >4.0 mU/L at the outset of screening, then thyroxine should be initiated. The evidence base is presently not strong with regard to thyroxine administration in this way reducing miscarriages but current guidelines suggest this to be appropriate (Figure 1.3).

Chlamydia trachomatis is present in more than 10% of the young sexually active population. It is a major cause of pelvic infection and the sequelae of pain, ectopic pregnancy and tubal factor infertility are well recognised. The prevalence of *C. trachomatis* in infertile women is less than 2% but uterine instrumentation may lead to upper genital tract spread of endocervical colonisation. This may lead to pelvic infection and tubal compromise in women with or without pre-existing tubal disease. Screening for *C. trachomatis* should be integral to the workup of the infertile woman and, if positive, treatment should be administered and appropriate specialist genitourinary medicine clinic referral made. Bacterial vaginosis may also be detected through screening and should be treated in symptomatic women or where uterine instrumentation is required.

The investigations outlined in the foregoing can be initiated by the GP but they also provide the basis for hospital investigation. It may be helpful to send the couple a questionnaire to supplement the information provided in the GP's referral letter. Valuable time can be saved if progesterone monitoring, evidence of rubella immunisation, *Chlamydia* screening and semen analysis are performed in line with current guidelines before referral to the fertility clinic.

In the specialist clinic setting a pelvic ultrasound examination will be useful. It may reveal potentially significant pathology, for example, fibroids, intrauterine polyps and ovarian cysts, which might be missed in bimanual pelvic examination. Assessment of the antral follicle count should be carried out. This measure of ovarian reserve may be particularly useful in women who have irregular/short cycles occasionally associated with premature ovarian insufficiency (POI). If there is a suspicion of POI on ultrasound it may be appropriate to test this further through measurement of anti-mullerian hormone (AMH). Low levels will reinforce the suspicion of POI and may influence the pace at which fertility treatment may be offered. A polycystic appearance of the ovaries may be found in normally cycling women as well as those with classic features of infrequent periods and signs of androgen excess. Tests of ovarian reserve will be discussed in more detail in Chapters 2 and 7.

1.5 General Advice for Practitioners to Give to Patients

Table 1.4 gives a summary of lifestyle advice which health professionals should provide to infertile patients. There is reasonable evidence to support the suggestion that smoking reduces female fertility, while in men it is known that smoking may affect sperm quality.

In men there is evidence that high alcohol intake can influence reproductive function adversely, as well

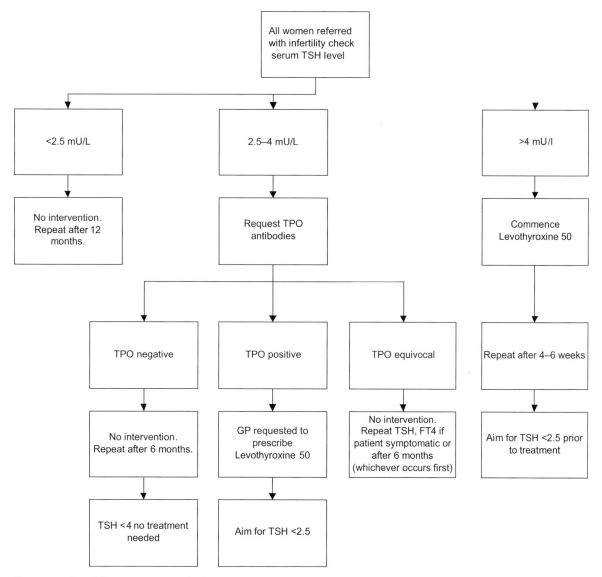

Figure 1.3 Thyroid function testing in infertility care.

as general health. A maximum of 3–4 units per day should be advised. There is less convincing evidence linking alcohol and female fertility, but intake in excess of 2 units per day of alcohol more than twice a week, as well as episodes of intoxication, should be discouraged.

There is no consistent evidence at the present time with respect to caffeine use and fertility in men and women. The use of recreational drugs including marijuana and cocaine may adversely affect ovulatory function and tubal function. Appropriate advice should be given.

Women with a body mass index in excess of 30 should be encouraged to lose weight as, in those with disturbed regulation of ovulation, this alone may restore normal function, or alternatively enhance the response to treatment where instituted.

While there is some evidence that sperm parameters may be adversely affected by very frequent ejaculation the evidence suggests that fertility potential is unaffected. Bearing in mind that sperm survival can be expected for up to 7 days within the female reproductive tract, couples should be advised to have intercourse every 2–3 days to optimise the chance of

Table 1.4 Summary of lifestyle advice given to patients

Advice	Action
Smoking	Advise both partners to stop.
Alcohol	Both partners need to limit alcohol intake if attempting to conceive.
BMI	Encourage women with a body mass index in excess of 30 to lose weight.
Sexual intercourse	Couples should be advised to have regular intercourse at least two or three times per week.

conception. Hyperthermia may adversely affect sperm quality and should be avoided.

1.6 Further Tests

1.6.1 Female

Where preliminary investigations suggest that the woman is ovulating and sperm production is satisfactory, pelvic assessment should be considered. For those with symptoms of painful periods or examination findings suggestive of pelvic pathology then laparoscopy and dye hydrotubation will be the investigation of choice. Endometriosis and peritubal adhesions may be found. If a suspicion of pelvic pathology is entertained before surgery then permission may be given for a 'see and treat' approach allowing simple measures, for example, ablation of endometriosis, adhesiolysis, ovarian cystectomy or tubal surgery, to be carried out during the 'diagnostic' procedure.

Hysterosalpingo-contrast sonography (HyCoSy) is an outpatient investigation which may be used to evaluate tubal patency. Similarly, an x-ray hysterosalpingogram (HSG) may also be used as a first-line examination in women with a low risk of pelvic pathology. Tubal assessment should not be carried out if the patient is menstruating. In addition, women should be advised to avoid conception in the cycle in which the procedure is carried out. If unprotected intercourse has occurred, then the examination should be deferred.

It is important to ensure that antibiotic treatment, for example, with azithromycin or doxycycline, is given at the time of uterine instrumentation to those women at risk of *Chlamydia* infection.

It is debatable whether assessment of tubal status is necessary in situations in which women present with long-standing, otherwise unexplained, infertility. Present evidence would suggest that minor abnormalities of the uterine cavity such as tubocornual polyps

may be of little importance in the genesis of infertility. Saline infusion sonography can facilitate visualisation of intrauterine and tubal pathology. Prospective studies are also awaited to determine whether hysteroscopy may have a part to play in the routine investigation of infertile women, though in women with identified intrauterine abnormalities hysteroscopic surgery may be feasible.

1.6.2 Male

The capacity of sperm to fertilise an egg depends on a complex series of biological events including transport to the site of fertilisation, sperm–egg recognition, the acrosome reaction and fusion of the sperm to the oocyte. Dispute remains with respect to the value of the post-coital test (PCT) in providing information about sperm function in the man. Review of the literature would suggest that the test lacks validity for routine use. Nevertheless, if sexual dysfunction is suspected, or the male partner cannot or will not provide a semen sample for analysis, the PCT may have a place, even at an early stage in investigation. It is crucial that the test is done at the correct stage in the cycle, that is, at the time of maximal cervical mucus production prior to ovulation. Inappropriate timing of the test may provide misleading information and cause unnecessary concern. Ideally, mucus production should be assessed daily using an objective method. Occasionally, mucus production may be poor until the day of the beginning of the LH surge and this may indicate a functional problem within the cervix, an unusual situation even in cases in which there has been previous cervical surgery. This need for precise timing leads to a sex-on-demand approach to investigation which may produce additional strain and tension for an already overburdened couple trying to cope with the stress of their infertility and their associated loss of self-esteem.

Other tests of sperm function including computerised analysis of sperm-movement characteristics and sperm cervical mucus penetration tests, DNA fragmentation, are not recommended for routine use, nor are the testing for anti-sperm antibodies in semen. The place for such tests will be discussed in Chapter 5.

1.7 Reaching a Diagnosis

The management of people with infertility problems is largely dictated by the major diagnostic category into which they fit. Typical figures are shown in Table 1.5.

Diagnostic categories in most studies include male factors, disorders of ovulation, tubal factors, endometriosis and uterine factor related infertility and unexplained infertility. When analysed, the distribution of causes will be affected by whether the woman has been pregnant in the past. The association in cases of secondary infertility with an increased risk of tubal factor infertility, however, should not lead to complacency in respect of the possibility that male factors may contribute to a couple's infertility even where the man has fathered a pregnancy in the past. It should be borne in mind that more than one factor may contribute to a couple's infertility and each may require simultaneous management, for example, ovulation induction for a woman who is not ovulating in combination with donor insemination.

1.8 Prognosis

It is generally accepted that the three most important factors determining the chance of natural or assisted conception in infertile individuals are the age of the female partner, the duration of infertility and whether there has been a conception previously. Once a diagnosis is reached any judgement on the prognosis for conception must take these issues into account. Initiating intrusive and potentially harmful treatment should take account of natural expectations of pregnancy. In addition, it is important in making a judgement about interventions to take into consideration the potential hazards of treatment for the female partner as well as considerations of potential harm to offspring. In many instances expectant management will be appropriate.

For male factor infertility, which accounts for up to 25% of cases, the impairment of fertility may be exaggerated if the female partner is in her advanced reproductive years. Some men with impaired fertility may not present to the fertility clinic if their partner is above average fertility herself.

Ovulatory disorders, often associated with irregular menstruation, are associated with reduced natural chances of pregnancy. Ovulation induction provides good chances of success assuming no other complicating factors such as tubal compromise or severe impairment in sperm quality. Significantly overweight women are less responsive to treatment. Women with ovarian insufficiency will have a very pessimistic outlook.

Tubal factor infertility, accounting for up to 30% of infertile individuals, may have profound effects on the natural chances of establishing pregnancy, particularly if severe pelvic distortion is present.

Unexplained infertility accounts for around a quarter of the couples seen in fertility clinics. Treatment-independent pregnancies are a particular issue in this group of patients in our evaluation of the cost-effectiveness of interventions. In younger patients with short duration of infertility expectant management will be appropriate. In older patients this may not be the best option.

These issues will be discussed in much greater detail in other chapters in this book.

1.9 Conclusion

The preliminary assessment of egg and sperm availability, together with a determination that the gametes can meet, should provide a diagnosis for the majority of couples. In most cases, a prognosis, often favourable, can be given to the couple. Appropriate therapeutic strategies can be instituted where required, with specialist involvement if necessary. The lines of communication within a regional framework should be set out clearly, with the involvement of GPs intimately linked to the process of assessment (see Chapter 14). Clinical protocols should be clearly set out in order that unnecessary repetition of investigations is minimised. Clinics should be structured so that the same practitioner sees patients as far as possible and if subspecialist help is required this should be readily available. Information leaflets are a valuable adjunct to the smooth running of the clinic and suitably trained nursing staff should be an integral part of the service, providing a day-to-day focus for patient contact. Such personnel can plan and co-ordinate treatment protocols on an individual basis and, linked

Table 1.5 Diagnostic categories and distribution of couples with primary and secondary infertility

Diagnostic category	Infertility	
	Primary (%)	Secondary (%)
Male factor	25	20
Disorders of ovulation	20	15
Tubal factor	15	40
Endometriosis	10	5
Unexplained	30	20

to a sympathetic counselling service, will be able to best serve the considerable and complex needs of the infertile population entrusted to their care.

****

References

1. Zegers-Hochschild F, Adamson GD, Dyer S, et al. The international glossary on infertility and fertility care. *Hum Reprod.* 2017;**32**:1786–1801.

2. Evers JL. Female subfertility. *Lancet* 2002;**360**:151–9.

3. Bhattacharya S, Porter M, Almaraj E, et al. The epidemiology of infertility in the North East of Scotland. *Hum Reproduction* 2009 **24** 3096–107.

4. National Institute for Clinical Excellence. Fertility problems: assessment and treatment. Clinical Guideline (CG156). www.nice.org.uk\\guidance\\cg156 (updates September 6, 2017).

5. WHO Laboratory. *Manual for the examination and processing of human semen*, 5th ed. Department of Reproductive Health and Research, World Health Organization; 2010.www.who.int\\reproductivehealth\\publications\\infertility/

Disorders of Ovulation and Reproductive Endocrine Disorders Associated with Infertility

Sesh K. Sunkara

2.1 Introduction

Infertility is defined as the inability to achieve a clinical pregnancy after 12 months of regular unprotected sexual intercourse. Infertility can result from male and female contributing factors, assessed as part of baseline infertility investigations, and disorders of ovulation account for nearly a quarter of all infertility cases. The World Health Organization (WHO) classifies ovulation disorders into three groups, based on the most common reasons for anovulatory infertility:

Group I: Hypothalamic–pituitary disorders (hypothalamic amenorrhoea or hypogonadotropic hypogonadism)

Group II: Hypothalamic–pituitary–ovarian dysfunction (predominately polycystic ovary syndrome)

Group III: Ovarian failure

Cyclic mono-follicular recruitment and ovulation occur as a result of a complex interaction of hormones secreted by the hypothalamus, pituitary and ovary. The hypothalamus secretes gonadotropin-releasing hormone (GnRH), a decapeptide released in a pulsatile manner which stimulates the anterior pituitary secretion of gonadotrophins: follicle-stimulating hormone (FSH) and luteinising hormone (LH). Through their action on the ovary, FSH and LH in turn facilitate follicular recruitment, maturation, ovulation and the various stages of the menstrual cycle. This chapter details the various ovulatory disorders and their fertility management, the most common cause being polycystic ovary syndrome. As good practice would dictate, it is important to ensure that other factors contributing to infertility are excluded or dealt with appropriately before ovulation induction treatment for ovulatory disorders.

2.2 WHO Group II: Polycystic Ovary Syndrome

Polycystic ovary syndrome (PCOS) is the most common female endocrine disorder and is responsible for approximately 75% of ovulatory disorders. It is a complex reproductive and metabolic disorder and was first described in 1935 as Stein–Leventhal syndrome. The aetiology of PCOS remains unclear and the variations in phenotype lead to challenges for clinical management. PCOS is associated with clinical manifestations and health implications during adolescence and the reproductive and post-reproductive stages of a woman's life. Quite a few definitions and criteria have been proposed for the diagnosis of PCOS, of which the most commonly endorsed is the 2003 Rotterdam consensus on diagnostic criteria for PCOS [1]. According to the Rotterdam criteria, the diagnosis of PCOS is based on the fulfilment of any two of the following three criteria: (1) oligo- or anovulation, (2) clinical and/or biochemical signs of hyperandrogenism and (3) polycystic ovaries (Figure 2.1) and exclusion of other aetiologies (congenital adrenal hyperplasia, androgen-secreting tumours, Cushing's syndrome).

Traditionally, the first-line management of women with PCOS has been weight management to optimise both reproductive and metabolic outcomes. Observational studies have reported pregnancies after loss of as little as 5% of initial body weight [2, 3]. Weight optimisation is also suggested to enhance outcomes of pharmacological and surgical ovulation induction treatments. However, recent studies have not been able to confirm the beneficial effects of weight loss and successful pregnancies in women with anovulatory PCOS [4]. Nonetheless, given the beneficial effects of weight loss in mitigating the adverse metabolic associations with PCOS and obesity, preconceptual weight optimisation is a useful

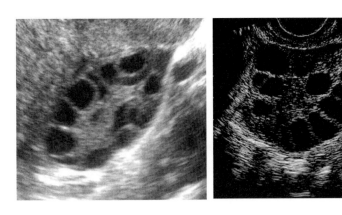

Figure 2.1 Transvaginal ultrasound appearance of polycystic ovaries.

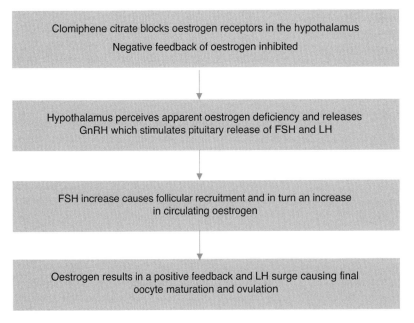

Figure 2.2 Mechanism of action of clomiphene citrate.

intervention. The following is an overview of the treatment options and treatment hierarchy for women with PCOS and anovulation.

2.2.1 Clomiphene Citrate for Ovulation Induction in PCOS

Clomiphene citrate (CC) is an anti-oestrogen which competes for receptor-binding sites with endogenous oestrogens. By blocking oestrogen receptors in the hypothalamus and pituitary, CC interferes with the feedback mechanism of endogenous oestrogen on the pituitary and hypothalamus. This results in an increase in FSH and LH secretion by the anterior pituitary, which stimulates ovarian follicular recruitment and ovulation (Figure 2.2). Clomiphene citrate has been used for ovulation induction in anovulatory women since the first published results on its application in 1961 [5].

There is evidence of a higher pregnancy and ovulation rate with CC compared to placebo or no treatment [6, 7]. Clomiphene citrate induces ovulation in 75%–80% of women [8, 9], with cumulative live birth rates of 50%–60% after six cycles [10]. The National Institute for Clinical Excellence (NICE) guidelines state that first-line pharmacological treatment for women with PCOS should be CC for up to six cycles [11]. They recommended a starting daily dose of CC of 50 mg for 5 days in the early phase of the menstrual cycle. If ovulation is not achieved with the lowest dose of 50 mg daily, the dose of CC can be increased in 50-mg increments to 100 mg, and ultimately a maximum of 150 mg daily. If ovulation is confirmed, treatment with CC can be continued for six cycles. Failure to ovulate after the maximum dose of 150 mg daily is termed CC resistance. Second-line ogvulation induction options should be considered in cases of CC resistance.

Clomiphene citrate can induce multiple follicular recruitment and is associated with a multiple pregnancy rate of around 10%. Clomiphene citrate has anti-oestrogenic effects on the endometrium which can result in a thin endometrium, although the implications are unclear [12]. Ultrasound monitoring, at least in the first cycle of treatment, is indicated to assess follicular recruitment and the endometrial thickness. Strict criteria (usually two or three follicles ≥14 mm based on female age) for cycle cancellation in case of multiple follicles should be established to reduce multiple pregnancies with CC therapy.

Tamoxifen is another anti-oestrogen that can be used for ovulation induction in WHO group II women. A Cochrane review on anti-oestrogen for ovulation induction for women with PCOS showed no significant differences between CC and tamoxifen for outcomes of live birth, clinical pregnancy and miscarriage. There were insufficient data to draw any conclusion regarding multiple pregnancies [6]. The dosage of tamoxifen varied from 10 mg to 60 mg daily among the studies included in the Cochrane review and pooled in the meta-analysis. There was no consistency in the duration of treatment.

2.2.2 Insulin-Sensitising Agents for Ovulation Induction in PCOS

Polycystic ovary syndrome is an insulin-resistant disorder characterised by hyperinsulinaemia (Figure 2.3). Increased insulin resistance, hyperandrogenism and obesity have a significant impact on menstrual cyclicity and reproductive health.

Metformin is an anti-hyperglycaemic biguanide and a commonly used insulin-sensitising drug. It is considered to be beneficial for women with PCOS for fertility and control of metabolic symptoms. The UK NICE guidelines (2013) recommend metformin alone or in combination with CC as first-line treatment for women with PCOS and anovulation on the basis of its insulin-sensitising property. However, the evidence for beneficial reproductive outcomes is not conclusive. The most recent Cochrane review on metformin versus placebo for ovulation induction in women with PCOS showed metformin to be associated with higher clinical pregnancy rates (odds ratio [OR] 1.93; 95% CI 1.42 to 2.64) and may improve live birth rates (OR 1.59; 95% CI 1.00 to 2.51) but the quality of evidence for the latter was low (13). When metformin plus CC was compared to CC alone, higher clinical pregnancy rates were found with the combined therapy compared to CC alone (OR 3.97; 95% CI 2.59 to 6.08). There was, however, no conclusive difference in live birth rates between metformin plus CC versus CC alone (OR 1.21; 95% CI 0.92 to 1.59) but the quality of evidence was low.

The recent WHO guidance on the management of anovulatory infertility in women with PCOS recommends metformin used alone if facilities are not available for monitoring of CC or letrozole, which are more effective. It also recommends metformin in combination with CC to improve fertility outcomes in women

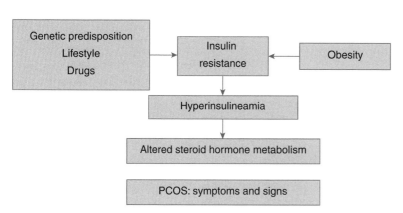

Figure 2.3 Insulin resistance contributing to PCOS symptoms.

with PCOS who are CC resistant [14]. Metformin is frequently associated with gastrointestinal side effects, which should be considered when prescribing.

2.2.3 Aromatase Inhibitors for Ovulation Induction in PCOS

Aromatase inhibitors were introduced for ovulation induction in 2001 [15]. They prevent aromatisation of androgens to oestrogens and this decrease in oestrogens releases the pituitary from the negative feedback effect, with a resulting increase in FSH that effects ovarian stimulation and follicular recruitment (Figure 2.4). A network meta-analysis of studies comparing the effectiveness of first-line ovulation induction treatment options for women with PCOS showed the aromatase inhibitor letrozole was the most effective treatment in terms of live birth [7]. Compared to CC alone, treatment with letrozole led to significantly higher ovulation (OR 1.99; 95% CI 1.38 to 2.87), pregnancy (OR 1.58; 95% CI 1.25 to 2.00) and live birth rates (OR 1.67; 95% CI 1.11 to 2.49) and significantly lower multiple pregnancy rates (OR 0.46; 95% CI 0.23 to 0.92). A recent updated Cochrane review on the use of letrozole as an ovulation induction agent showed a higher live birth rate with letrozole compared to CC (OR 1.68; 95% CI 1.42 to 1.99). The UK NICE guidance on fertility which was updated before this evidence does not recommend letrozole for ovulation induction. However, other recent guidelines such as the WHO [14] and International PCOS guideline [16] recommend letrozole use for ovulation induction in women with PCOS.

2.2.4 Ovarian Drilling for Ovulation Induction in PCOS

Surgical ovarian wedge resection, first performed by Stein and Leventhal in 1935 and carried out via laparotomy, was a treatment for women with anovulatory PCOS but was largely abandoned both due to the risk of post-surgical adhesions and the introduction of medical ovulation induction. However, not all ovulation induction medications are successful in inducing ovulation and ovarian surgery continues to be a second-line treatment option. The advent of laparoscopy has facilitated laparoscopic ovarian drilling (LOD) which can be performed with fewer post-operative side effects over open surgery. In the current set-ups LOD can be performed as day case procedures, making it more cost effective. The UK NICE guideline recommends LOD as a treatment option for CC-resistant PCOS. The endocrine changes following surgery are also thought to convert the adverse androgen-dominant intrafollicular environment to an oestrogenic one and to restore the hormonal environment to normal by correcting disturbances of the ovarian–pituitary feedback mechanism [17].

Both local and systemic effects are thought to promote follicular recruitment, maturation and subsequent ovulation following LOD in women with PCOS and anovulation. The rationale is to destroy ovarian androgen-producing tissue and reduce the peripheral conversion of androgens to oestrogens. The fall in serum oestrogens causes a resultant rise in FSH which stimulates the ovaries and promotes follicular recruitment. The Cochrane review comparing gonadotropins with LOD in women with CC-resistant PCOS found that there was no difference between the two options in terms of live birth rate, long-term cost and quality of life. Laparoscopic ovarian drilling was associated with significantly lower multiple pregnancy rate compared to gonadotropins (OR 0.13; 95% CI 0.03 to 0.52) and short-term treatment costs ($P < 0.00001$) [18]. In addition to CC-resistant PCOS, LOD may be useful for women who are unable to comply with the intensive

Figure 2.4 Mechanism of action of aromatase inhibitors.

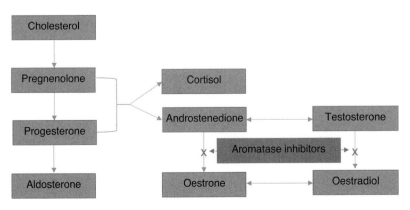

ultrasound monitoring needed with gonadotropin treatment. The minimum effective (intervention/dose) should be used for ovarian drilling to achieve ovulation and minimise the risk of ovarian damage and potential effect on ovarian reserve. There is inconsistent evidence on the minimum effective (intervention/dose) to achieve ovulation and minimise the risk of ovarian damage when using LOD, and the potential effect on ovarian reserve requires further investigation [14].

2.2.5 Gonadotrophins for Ovulation Induction in PCOS

Use of gonadotrophins for ovulation induction is indicated in women who have failed to conceive despite evidence of ovulation following alternative treatments or in women with CC-resistant PCOS. This strategy is potentially associated with a high risk of multiple pregnancy, which necessitates intensive ultrasound monitoring and strict cycle cancellation criteria. The aim is to achieve successful unifollicular ovulation and avoid multiple pregnancy as well as ovarian hyperstimulation syndrome (OHSS).

Treatment strategies such as the step-up regime, step-down regime and low-dose step-up regimes have been advocated to enhance the effectiveness of gonadotropin ovulation induction with minimal side effects (Figure 2.5).

The commonly used low-dose step-up regimen employs a starting dose of 50–75 IU daily which is increased only after 14 days if there is no response and then by only 25–37.5 IU every 7 days [19]. Ovulation is usually triggered with a single injection of 5000 units of human chorionic gonadotropin (hCG) when at least one follicle of at least 17 mm in its largest diameter has developed. To reduce the risks of multiple pregnancy and OHSS, hCG should not be administered in the presence of three or more follicles larger than 14 mm in diameter.

In overstimulated cycles, hCG is withheld and the patient is counselled about the risks and advised to refrain from sexual intercourse. An ovulation induction strategy applying CC as first-line treatment and gonadotropins as second-line treatment is associated with live birth rates of around 75%–80% [20].

An summary of this approach to ovulation induction in PCOS is shown in Figure 2.6. If ovulation induction treatments are unsuccessful or if there are other infertility factors such as a contributing male or tubal factor, in vitro fertilisation (IVF) treatment should be considered for the treatment of infertility in women with PCOS. It is important to consider the important challenges that are associated with assisted reproductive technology and treatments tailored accordingly. This is explored further in Chapter 7.

Gonadotropin Therapy

Figure 2.5 Gonadotropin treatment regimes.

- Conventional step-up
  - Starting does 75IU
  - Increase by 75IU after 7 days
  - Increase every 3-5 days until response
- Low-dose step-up
  - Start with 37.5–75IU
  - Do not increase for 14 days
  - 25-37.5IU increments every 7 days until threshold
- Step-down
  - Decrease dose when follicle recruited
  - Decrease again 3days later until day of hCG

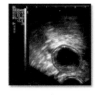
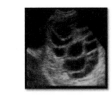

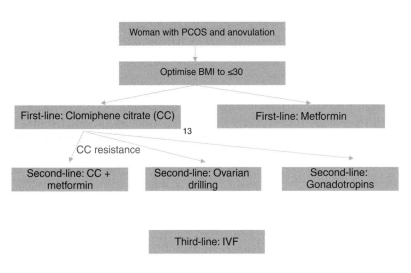

Figure 2.6 Ovulation induction for women with PCOS: approach as per NICE (2013) guidance.

2.3 WHO Group I: Hypothalamic and Pituitary Disorders of Anovulation

Hypothalamic–pituitary, WHO group 1 disorders, cause hypogonadotropic hypogonadism resulting in anovulatory infertility. These include pituitary disorders such as hyperprolactinaemia, Kallmann syndrome and functional hypothalamic amenorrhoea (caused by weight loss, stress or excessive exercise).

2.3.1 Hyperprolactinaemia

Prolactin (PRL) is secreted by pituitary lactotroph cells and its prime function is to induce and maintain lactation of the primed breast. Non-puerperal hyperprolactinaemia is caused by lactotroph adenomas (prolactinomas), which account for approximately 40% of all pituitary tumours. Hyperprolactinaemia may also develop due to pharmacological or pathological interruption of hypothalamic–pituitary dopaminergic pathways and is sometimes idiopathic. A serum PRL level above the upper limit of normal confirms the diagnosis of hyperprolactinaemia as long as the serum sample is obtained without excessive venipuncture stress. A single determination is usually sufficient but when in doubt, repeat sampling is suggested. Regardless of aetiology, hyperprolactinaemia may result in hypogonadism, infertility and galactorrhoea.

2.3.1.1 Causes of Hyperprolactinaemia

Hyperprolactinaemia comprises two types: functional or organic. The most common causes of functional mild to moderate hyperprolactinaemia are a variety of pharmacotherapeutic agents that reduce hypothalamic secretion of dopamine or its action in the pituitary such as certain anti-depressants (phenothiazines, haloperidol, risperidone, reserpine), anti-psychotics (monoamine oxidase inhibitors, selective serotonin reuptake inhibitors, tricyclic and tetracyclic agents), anti-emetics (metoclopramide, domperidone), opiates (morphine, methadone) and drugs such as cocaine.

Prolactin is a single globular polypeptide hormone, synthesised and secreted by pituitary lactotroph cells. It exists in heterogeneous sizes in serum, with three major variants: monomeric, dimeric and polymeric isoforms. Prolactin is synthesised as a prehormone, and after cleavage, the resulting hormone is a monomeric isoform of PRL. Monomeric PRL is the major form in the blood of subjects with normoprolactinaemia and true hyperprolactinaemia, accounting for 80%–95% of the total PRL. The other forms of PRL include the dimeric and polymeric isoforms and macroprolactin. The term 'macroprolactinaemia' is characterised by the predominance of macroprolactin, and it is suspected mainly in asymptomatic subjects or those without typical hyperprolactinaemia-related symptoms [21].

Functional hyperprolactinaemia is typically observed in pregnancy but it often occurs in PCOS, renal failure, hepatic cirrhosis and renal and lung cancers. Pathological functional hyperprolactinaemia also recurs in endocrinopathies such as primary hypothyroidism and primary adrenocortical insufficiency [22, 23]. In addition, mild stress, including that of venipuncture, can induce transient elevations in serum PRL.

Organic hyperprolactinaemia is mainly due to sellar and parasellar lesions, including pituitary adenomas (prolactinoma, PRL-secreting adenomas). In women, microadenomas (<1 cm in size) are more common than macroadenomas (>1 cm in size). Non-pituitary tumours and infiltrative conditions (such as sarcoidosis, craniopharyngioma, empty sella syndrome, vascular malformations, pituitary metastases or non-functioning adenomas compressing the pituitary stalk) frequently cause raised serum PRL levels through a disconnection that interrupts the normal dopaminergic inhibition of lactotroph cells [24].

2.3.1.2 Diagnosis and Treatment of Hyperprolactinaemia

A good medical history to exclude physiological, pharmacological and pathological causes of hyperprolactinaemia is important. In addition to serum PRL measurement, radiological imaging by MRI to identify pituitary tumours should be undertaken as indicated to establish the diagnosis and delineate the cause of hyperprolactinaemia.

The ideal treatment for patients with functional asymptomatic hyperprolactinaemia is removal of the relevant cause, for example, stopping or changing medication, reducing stress levels if likely contributory, weight gain if BMI is less than 19 kg/m^2 and avoiding excessive exercise. Medical therapy is the first choice in patients with prolactinomas and consists of use of dopamine agonists as first-line treatment to reduce tumour size and PRL levels. In patients with asymptomatic ovulatory microprolactinoma, no treatment needs to be given and a regular follow-up with serial PRL measurements and pituitary imaging should be organised. The majority of patients with prolactinomas, both micro- and macro-prolactinomas, can be successfully treated with dopamine agonists, with normalisation of PRL secretion and gonadal function, and significant tumour shrinkage in a high percentage of cases. The most commonly used dopamine agonists are bromocriptine and cabergoline. Cabergoline, because of its pharmacodynamics, has better tolerability and efficacy comparable to that of bromocriptine. Cabergoline normalises PRL levels and decreases tumour size, restoring gonadal function in 95% of microprolactinomas and 80% of macroprolactinomas, generally at the median dose of 0.5 mg per week and 1 mg per week, respectively. Bromocriptine has the longest history of use and is a safe, inexpensive and effective therapy option, with the therapeutic doses in the range of 2.5–15 mg per day (median: 7.5 mg). Doses as high as 20–30 mg per day may be necessary in approximately 30% of patients. However, bromocriptine requires multiple daily dosing and some patients are resistant or intolerant to this therapy because of side effects such as nausea, headache, constipation and nasal congestion. If PRL levels are well controlled with dopamine agonists, gradual tapering of the dose to the lowest effective amount is recommended, and sometimes medication can be stopped after several years. Trans-sphenoidal surgical resection of the prolactinoma remains the main option for patients who may refuse or do not respond to long-term pharmacological therapy [25].

2.3.2 Hypogonadotropic Hypogonadism

Hypothalamic–pituitary failure manifests as hypogonadotropic hypogonadism. Females with primary hypothalamic–pituitary failure typically present with delayed or impaired pubertal development, primary or secondary amenorrhoea and infertility. Idiopathic hypogonadotropic hypogonadism due to a congenital absence of GnRH is the most common cause of hypothalamic–pituitary failure. Idiopathic hypogonadotropic hypogonadism associated with anosmia is termed Kallmann syndrome, which results from failure of GnRH neuronal migration from the olfactory placode during embryonic development. Acquired causes include panhypopituitarism caused by tissue necrosis (secondary to acute ischemia or pituitary gland apoplexy), autoimmune or infectious hypophysitis and compression by pituitary adenomas or adjacent brain tumours. Sheehan syndrome is an example of acquired panhypopituitarism as a consequence of severe obstetric haemorrhage [26].

2.3.2.1 Diagnosis and Treatment

Diagnosis of hypogonadotropic hypogonadism is made from a history of amenorrhoea (primary or secondary), basal levels of FSH and LH accompanied by low serum oestradiol levels and a hypo-oestrogenic state. Fertility treatment involves either physiological correction of the hypogonadotropic state with pulsatile administration of GnRH or ovulation induction with gonadotropins such as human menopausal gonadotropin (hMG). As these women lack endogenous LH, it is important to give gonadotropins that have LH activity for successful ovulation induction. Administration of pulsatile GnRH requires a special pump that might not be available in all setting but has the advantage of physiological uni-follicular recruitment. Use of gonadotropins for ovulation induction has the disadvantage of inducing multiple follicles, resulting in multiple pregnancies, and hence should have stringent criteria for monitoring both to observe successful follicular recruitment and at the same time cancellation criteria in case of multifollicular recruitment along the lines described earlier for the use of gonadotropins for women with PCOS.

2.4 WHO Group III: Premature Ovarian Insufficiency

Premature ovarian insufficiency (POI) is a result of ovarian failure and is classified under WHO group III ovulation disorders. POI is a clinical syndrome defined by loss of ovarian activity before the age of 40 years. POI is characterised by menstrual disturbance (amenorrhoea or oligomenorrhoea) with raised gonadotropin levels and low oestradiol. The prevalence of POI is approximately 1%. The diagnosis POI is based on the presence of menstrual disturbance (oligo/amenorrhoea for at least 4 months) and biochemical confirmation (FSH level >25 IU/L on two occasions 4 weeks apart)[27].

Diagnosis of POI is made from a history of amenorrhoea, high levels of FSH and LH accompanied by low serum oestradiol levels and a hypo-oestrogenic state. POI is a hypergonadotropic hypogonadal state. It can result from genetic causes (e.g. Turner syndrome, fragile X premutation, autoimmune causes (associated, not clearly delineated), iatrogenic causes (surgery, chemotherapy and radiotherapy). However, the majority of cases of POI remain idiopathic with no delineated cause.

Premature ovarian insufficiency has both reproductive and general health implications, such as cardiovascular disorders and reduced bone mineral density. Oestrogen replacement therapy should be considered to alleviate the symptoms and health consequences from the hypo-oestrogenic state. Women should be informed that there is a very small chance of natural conception due to sporadic ovulation. Women wishing to conceive should therefore avoid the combined contraceptive pill (COCP) for oestrogen supplementation. Hormone replacement therapy (HRT) would be ideal in such women. Oocyte donation is the fertility treatment option for women with POI. In certain conditions such as Turner syndrome assessment and preconceptional specialist assessment should be considered to anticipate and mitigate obstetric complications.

2.5 Summary and Conclusions

Anovulation represents one of the main causes of female infertility, and establishing the underlying cause is critical to ensure effective treatment. A number of targeted interventions are available, ranging from lifestyle measures, oral medication, injectable hormones and assisted reproduction. The treatment strategy needs to take into account other co-existing factors and place equal emphasis on efficacy as well as safety.

References

1. Rotterdam ESHRE/ASRM-Sponsored PCOS Consensus Workshop Group. Revised 2003 consensus on diagnostic criteria and long-term health risks related to polycystic ovary syndrome. *Fertil Steril*. 2003;**81**:19–25.

2. Huber-Buchholz MM, Carey DG, Norman RJ. Restoration of reproductive potential by lifestyle modification in obese polycystic ovary syndrome: role of insulin sensitivity and luteinizing hormone. *J Clin Endocrinol Metab*. 1999;**84**:1470–4.

3. Kiddy DS, Hamilton-Fairley D, Bush A, Short F, Anyaoku V, Reed MJ, Franks S. Improvement in endocrine and ovarian function during dietary treatment of obese women with polycystic ovary syndrome. *Clin Endocrinol (Oxf)*. 1992;**36**:105–11.

4. Moran LJ, Hutchison SK, Norman RJ, Teede HJ. Lifestyle changes in women with polycystic ovary syndrome. *Cochrane Database Syst Rev*. 2011 Jul **6**;7:CD007506.

5. Greenblatt RB, Barfield WE, Jungck EC, Ray AW. Induction of ovulation with MRL/41: preliminary report. *JAMA*. 1961;**178**:101–4.

6. Brown J, Farquhar C. Clomiphene and other antioestrogens for ovulation induction in polycystic ovarian syndrome. *Cochrane Database Syst Rev*. 2016 Dec **15**;12:CD002249.

7. Wang R, Kim BV, van Wely M, et al. Treatment strategies for women with WHO group II anovulation: systematic review and network meta-analysis. *BMJ*. 2017;**31**:356:j138.

8. Homburg R. Clomiphene citrate: End of an era? A mini-review. *Hum Reprod*. 2005;**20**:2043–51.

9. Messinis IE. Ovulation induction: a mini review. *Hum Reprod*. 2005;**20**:2688–97.

10. Kousta E, White DM, Franks S. Modern use of clomiphene citrate in induction of ovulation. *Hum Reprod Update*. 1997;**3**:359–65.

11. NICE Clinical Guideline 156. Assessment and treatment for people with fertility problems. www .nice.org.uk\\guidance\\cg156

12. Gadalla MA, Huang S, Wang R, et al. Effect of clomiphene citrate on endometrial thickness, ovulation, pregnancy and live birth in anovulatory women: systematic review and meta-analysis. *Ultrasound Obstet Gynecol*. 2018;**51**:64–76.

13. Morley LC, Tang T, Yasmin E, Norman RJ, Balen AH. Insulin-sensitising drugs (metformin, rosiglitazone, pioglitazone, D-chiro-inositol) for women with polycystic ovary syndrome, oligo amenorrhoea and subfertility. *Cochrane Database Syst Rev*. 2017 Nov 29;11:CD003053.

14. Balen AH, Morley LC, Misso M, et al. The management of anovulatory infertility in women with polycystic ovary syndrome: an analysis of the evidence to support the development of global WHO guidance. *Hum Reprod Update*. 2016;**22**:687–708.

15. Mitwally MF, Casper RF. Use of an aromatase inhibitor for induction of ovulation in patients with an inadequate response to clomiphene citrate. *Fertil Steril*. 2001;**75**:305–9.

16. Teede HJ, Misso ML, Costello MF, et al.; International PCOS Network. Recommendations from the international evidence-based guideline for the assessment and management of polycystic ovary syndrome. *Hum Reprod*. 2018;**33**:1602–18.

17. Balen A, Tan SL, Jacobs H. Hypersecretion of luteinising hormone: a significant cause of infertility and miscarriage. *Br J Obstet Gynaecol*. 1993;**100**:1082–9.

18. Farquhar C, Brown J, Marjoribanks J. Laparoscopic drilling by diathermy or laser for ovulation induction in anovulatory polycystic ovary syndrome. *Cochrane Database Syst Rev*. 2012 Jun 13;6:CD001122.

19. White DM, Polson DW, Kiddy D, et al. Induction of ovulation with low-dose gonadotropins in polycystic ovary syndrome: an analysis of 109 pregnancies in 225 women. *J Clin Endocrinol Metab*. 1996;**81**:3821–4.

20. Veltman-Verhulst SM, van Haeften TW, Eijkemans MJ, de Valk HW, Fauser BC, Goverde AJ. Sex hormone-binding globulin concentrations before conception as a predictor for gestational diabetes in women with polycystic ovary syndrome. *Hum Reprod*. 2010;**25**:3123–8.

21. Kasum M, Pavičić-Baldani D, Stanić P, Orešković S, Sarić JM, Blajić J, Juras J. Importance of macroprolactinemia in hyperprolactinemia. *Eur J Obstet Gynecol Reprod Biol*. 2014 Dec;**183**:28–32.

22. Cortet-Rudelli C, Sapin R, Bonnecille JF, Brune T. Etiological diagnosis of hyperprolactinemia. *Ann Endocrinol (Paris)*. 2007;**68**:98–105.

23. Robin G, Catteau-Jonard S, Young J. Physiopathological link between polycystic ovary syndrome and hyperprolactinemia: myth or reality? *Gynecol Obstet Fertil*. 2011;**39**:141–5.

24. Verhelst J, Abs R. Hyperprolactinemia: pathophysiology and management. *Treat Endocrinol*. 2003;**2**:23–32.

25. Capozzi A, Scambia G, Pontecorvi A, Lello S. Hyperprolactinemia: pathophysiology and therapeutic approach. *Gynecol Endocrinol*. 2015;**31**:506–10.

26. Mikhael S, Punjala-Patel A, Gavrilova-Jordan L. Hypothalamic-pituitary-ovarian axis disorders impacting female fertility. *Biomedicines*. 2019;**7**. pii: E5.

27. European Society for Human Reproduction and Embryology (ESHRE) Guideline Group on POI, Webber L, Davies M, et al. ESHRE Guideline: management of women with premature ovarian insufficiency. *Hum Reprod*. 2016;**31**:926–37.

Chapter 3

Endometriosis

Lucky Saraswat

Endometriosis is a chronic gynaecological condition classically associated with dysmenorrhoea, pelvic pain and infertility, though some women can be asymptomatic. It is characterised by the presence and proliferation of endometrium-like tissue (glands and stroma) in ectopic sites outside the physiologically normal location of the uterine cavity [1]. The diagnosis is established by direct visualisation of lesions at laparoscopy.

3.1 Prevalence

Lack of pathognomonic signs and symptoms of endometriosis combined with the need for laparoscopy to confirm the diagnosis make it challenging to estimate the disease burden. The true prevalence of endometriosis in the general population hence remains unknown, although estimates range between 2% and 10% in women of reproductive age group [2]. The prevalence of endometriosis is significantly higher in women with pelvic pain or infertility, with reported rates varying between 20% and 50%. In a study of women undergoing laparoscopic sterilisation, the authors reported a 7% prevalence rate of endometriotic lesions in multiparous women. A multicentre Italian study [3] surveyed the prevalence of endometriosis in 3,684 women with selected gynaecological conditions requiring surgery. They reported that co-existing endometriosis was identified in 30% of women with infertility, 45% of women with pelvic pain, 35% of women with ovarian cysts and 12% of women with fibroids.

3.2 Aetiopathogenesis of Endometriosis

Several plausible theories regarding pathogenesis of endometriosis exist: some propose the origin of endometriosis from the uterine endometrium while others suggest an extrauterine origin for endometriotic implants. An increasing number of studies suggest an interplay of genetic, hormonal, environmental, immunological and oxidative factors in the development of endometriosis in susceptible women.

3.2.1 Hypotheses

The classical theories of pathogenesis are:

1. **Retrograde Menstruation (Sampson's Theory)**
   This is one of the most widely recognised theories for the genesis of endometriosis. In 1927, Sampson proposed the novel idea that ectopic endometrial tissue in the pelvis arises as a result of retrograde menstrual flow from the fallopian tubes into the abdominopelvic cavity. Presence of blood in the pelvis has been observed at surgical procedures in women during their menses. Animal models have confirmed that shed endometrial tissue has the ability to establish and grow outside the uterine cavity. The incidence of endometriosis is also higher in women with congenital anomalies associated with outflow tract obstruction that increase retrograde menstruation, such as an imperforate hymen or cervical stenosis.

2. **Metaplastic Transformation (Meyer's Theory)**
   Meyer proposed that endometriotic cells in the peritoneum originate from metaplasia of coelomic epithelium as a result of unknown stimuli. This is plausible, as both the peritoneum and endometrium share a common embryonic precursor, the coelomic cell. This theory may explain the occurrence of endometriosis in women who have had a hysterectomy and even in men undergoing oestrogen therapy.
   The 'induction theory' is an extension of the coelomic metaplasia theory and proposes that one or several endogenous, biochemical, or immunological factors may induce endometrial differentiation of undifferentiated cells.

3. **Lymphatic or Haematogenous Spread (Halban's Theory)** Halban proposed that endometriotic tissue can disseminate from the uterus to distant and extrapelvic sites through the lymphatic or vascular systems. This theory provides an explanation for cases in which endometriosis is found in remote sites such as the brain or pleura, but does not explain the mechanisms that allow cells to establish and proliferate in these extrapelvic sites.

4. **Direct Transplantation Theory** According to this theory, endometrial cells may become incorporated at surgical sites (e.g. at the site of an episiotomy or a caesarean section) during tissue trauma or surgical procedures. The initiation of a localised oncogenic-like cascade and lack of immunological response may result in implant survival.

5. **Theory of Mullerianosis**: This theory purports that the embryonic mullerian rests retain the capacity to develop into endometriotic lesions under hormonal (oestrogen) and environmental influences.

   More recently, differentiation of bone marrow stem cell lineages, such as mesenchymal or endothelial stem cells, into endometriosis has been proposed.

It is likely that various innate and acquired factors, such as genetics or environmental or immunological factors, acting in conjunction lead to the development of endometriosis in susceptible women. The different theories and mechanisms for the pathogenesis of endometriosis are depicted in Figure 3.1.

3.2.2 Genetic Factors

Endometriosis is inherited in a polygenic manner. Several candidate genes have been implicated. Some of these genes encode detoxification enzymes and thus may increase susceptibility to environmental stimuli. Other explanations include an abnormal epigenetic signature in the eutopic endometrium of women with endometriosis, which creates an altered hormonal milieu and an increase in the local concentration of oestrogen, thereby promoting development of ectopic implants.

3.2.3 Immunological Processes

The peritoneal environment in most women is capable of resorbing menstrual debris at the end of menstruation. In women with endometriosis, constitutional or acquired anomalies in endometrial cells evade immune clearance, conferring a survival advantage. Dysregulation of cell mediated immunity, increased endometrial autoantibodies, higher levels of cytokines and activation of lymphocytes and macrophages have been observed in the peritoneal fluid of women with endometriosis. Decreased cytotoxicity allows the shed

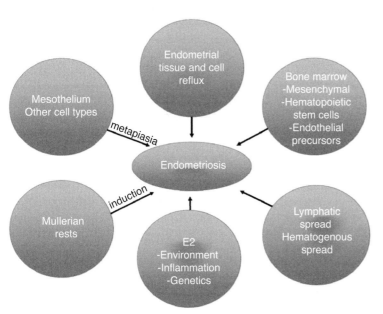

Figure 3.1 Theories of endometriosis pathogenesis.
Reproduced with permission from [1].

endometrial tissue to establish itself, while activated macrophages produce a higher amount of cytokines and growth factors, promoting disease progression through neuroangiogenesis and vasculogenesis. Endometriosis is frequently associated with extensive peritoneal adhesions. There is evidence to suggest that this may be a result of an impaired fibrinolytic system.

3.3 Disease Description, Distribution and Classification

Endometriotic lesions can be divided into three main types: peritoneal endometriosis, ovarian endometrioma and deep infiltrating endometriosis.

Peritoneal Endometriosis Peritoneal lesions are the most diverse in their morphological appearance and are classified as red (red, red-pink and clear), black (black and blue) and white (white, yellow-brown and peritoneal defects) lesions [4]. Atypical and subtle lesions are also common, presenting as serous or clear vesicular implants. Clinical evidence suggests that these appearances represent different stages of peritoneal lesions, with temporal progression of lesions from red vesicular to blue-black powder burn to fibrotic with adhesional changes. Defects in the pelvic peritoneum, or lacunae, referred to as Allen–Masters windows, may arise secondary to adhesion formation from the cyclical inflammatory changes associated with the endometriotic lesions.

Endometrioma Ovarian involvement typically presents as cysts progressively increasing in size and filled with chocolate coloured fluid – often referred to as 'chocolate cysts' or ovarian endometrioma classically adherent to pelvic side wall and the posterior aspect of uterus.

Deep Endometriosis Deep endometriosis is characterised by nodules extending more than 5 mm beneath the peritoneum and may involve the uterosacral ligaments, vagina, bowel, bladder or ureters. The depth of infiltration often correlates better with the type and severity of symptoms such as dyspareunia and dyschezia.

The common phenotypic subtypes of peritoneal endometriosis and ovarian endometrioma and deep endometriosis are illustrated in Figures 3.2 and 3.3.

Endometriotic lesions are predominantly confined to the abdominopelvic cavity in the pelvic peritoneum, ovaries, uterosacral ligaments or rectovaginal septum. Extrapelvic locations include surgical scars and the diaphragm or lungs, although other rare locations are possible. The anatomical distribution of endometriotic lesions is not even, with evidence of abdominopelvic,

anterior–posterior and left–right asymmetry [5]. They are more common in the pelvis than in the abdomen and have a predilection towards the pelvic cul-de-sac (the lowest part of the pelvis). This preferential location appears to be the result of the influence of gravity. Endometriosis is more common in the posterior compartment of the pelvis than the anterior compartment and in the left hemipelvis compared to the right. This distribution can be explained by the trajectory and direction of peritoneal flow and areas of stagnation of peritoneal fluid.

Endometriosis Classification The extent of the disease varies, from a few, small peritoneal lesions on otherwise normal pelvic organs, to large, ovarian endometrioma, adhesions or deep disease involving the uterosacral ligaments, large bowel and ureters, causing marked distortion of the pelvic anatomy. The best-known classification system for endometriosis is the revised American Society for Reproductive Medicine (r-ASRM) classification (1997). Depending on the extent and location of the disease, r-ASRM have classified endometriosis into four stages: minimal, mild, moderate, and severe, or stage I to IV. Other emerging systems include the Enzian classification for deep endometriosis and the endometriosis fertility index (EFI). All these classification systems have attracted criticism because of the poor correlation with disease symptoms as well as a lack of predictive prognosis for pain or infertility or response to treatment. The r-ASRM has been the oldest and most used system, though EFI has a better prognostic value for pregnancy rates because the latter includes clinical variables in addition to the surgical findings in the clinical scoring.

3.4 Epidemiology and Risk Factors

The majority of the risk factors for endometriosis relate to the concept that endometriosis is an oestrogen-dependent condition, associated with reflux of menstrual effluent into the peritoneal cavity [6].

Age Endometriosis is typically found in women of reproductive age with the peak age for diagnosis being 25–29 years. The age of onset is likely to be earlier as there is usually a significant delay between a woman's first presentation to primary care and a confirmed diagnosis of endometriosis. This interval has been reported to be around 8 years in the United Kingdom.

Menstrual and Reproductive Factors Early menarche (age <12 years), a short interval between cycles

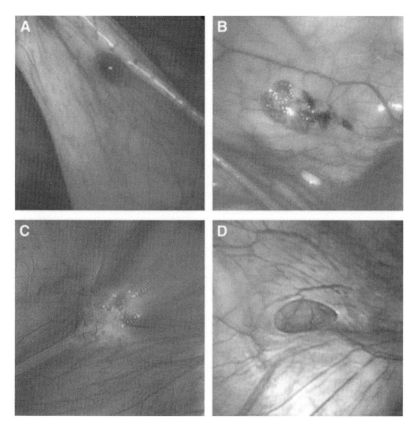

Figure 3.2 Phenotypic subtypes of peritoneal endometriosis. Reproduced with permission from [1].

and heavy menstrual flow have been consistently shown to be associated with an increased risk of endometriosis. This is related to increased exposure to menstrual efflux, strongly supporting Sampson's theory.

Dysmenorrhoea has a very strong link with endometriosis. Up to 50% of adolescent girls with severe dysmenorrhoea are diagnosed with endometriosis. Dysmenorrhoea may well be considered a symptom of the disease. An alternative explanation, that dysmenorrhoea is likely to be associated with some degree of outflow obstruction and a higher propensity to retrograde menstruation, potentially allows dysmenorrhoea to be classed as an independent risk factor for the development of endometriosis.

Association with parity is more complex, as infertility may be either a consequence or cause of the disease. An inverse association of endometriosis with parity is well established. Pregnancy and lactation are associated with a period of amenorrhoea, reducing exposure to menstrual endometrium. High progesterone levels present in pregnancy inhibit the establishment and growth of endometriotic deposits.

Race, Ethnicity and Social Class There is a non-validated clinical impression that endometriosis may vary with race, with black women having a lower rate of endometriosis and South-East Asian women having a higher rate than Caucasian women. A higher frequency of endometriosis is reported among women of higher social class. This may be influenced by diagnostic bias resulting from increased health awareness and better access to health care.

Smoking, Diet and Lifestyle Factors There is some evidence that smoking has a protective effect on endometriosis due to its anti-oestrogenic effect. Smoke compounds impair oestradiol and progesterone synthesis. Smoking, on the other hand, is proinflammatory and can trigger inflammation associated with endometriosis. A meta-analysis of 38 studies did not support any link between smoking and the risk of endometriosis [7]. Moderate alcohol consumption has been found to increase the risk of endometriosis. This effect is mediated through an increase in oestrogen levels secondary to increased aromatase activity or the impact of alcohol on release of luteinising hormone (LH) from the

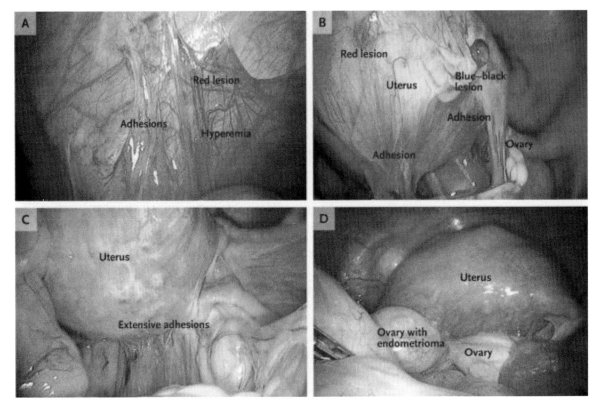

Figure 3.3 Peritoneal endometriosis, ovarian endometrioma and adhesions.

pituitary. A recent meta-analysis demonstrated a 1.2 times higher risk of endometriosis in women with regular alcohol intake compared to those who did not consume alcohol, with evidence supporting an argument for a dose-dependent relationship [8]. Data on the link between caffeine and endometriosis are insufficient. Caffeine inhibits aromatase, thereby reducing conversion of androgens to oestrogen. A protective effect of caffeine on endometriosis risk has not yet been confirmed.

Regular exercise or physical activity confers a protective effect on endometriosis by decreasing oestrogen production, reducing the levels of bio-available oestrogen by an increase in levels of serum hormone binding globulin (SHBG) and increasing systemic levels of anti-inflammatory cytokines. The positive effect of exercise on the reduced risk of endometriosis has been noted in a number of studies, although bias introduced through study design and selection of controls limits definitive interpretation.

Constitutional and Genetic Factors A literature review identified a modest, inverse relationship between adult BMI and risk of endometriosis. Likewise, taller women have higher follicular phase oestradiol and thereby a higher incidence of endometriosis.

Familial aggregation of endometriosis has been noted in population-based samples and twin studies. An up to six-fold increase in the risk of endometriosis is noted in the first-degree relatives of affected women with a polygenic pattern of inheritance. A strong familial tendency in non-human primates lends further support for a genetic predisposition.

3.5 Diagnosis of Endometriosis

3.5.1 Symptoms and Signs of Endometriosis

The two main characteristics of endometriosis are pain and infertility. Under the influence of oestrogen, ectopic endometrial implants are believed to undergo cyclical proliferation and shedding, causing an inflammatory response. This response is accompanied by angiogenesis, adhesions, fibrosis, neuronal infiltration and anatomical distortion resulting in pain and infertility or both.

The classical pain symptoms are dysmenorrhea (painful periods), chronic pelvic pain and deep dyspareunia (painful intercourse) [2, 9]. Other symptoms include cyclical intestinal complaints, dyschezia (pain when moving bowels) and fatigue. Symptoms tend to be cyclical but can occur at other times through the month. A proportion of women with the disease are asymptomatic. There is also a distinct lack of correlation between severity of symptoms and extent of the disease. The anatomic location and the depth of invasion appear to be more predictive than the area affected by endometriosis.

Endometriosis is identified in up to 40% of infertile women [2] and may be the only symptom in some. Several mechanisms have been postulated to explain the cause of infertility in women with endometriosis. In moderate to severe disease, extensive scarring and distortion of the pelvic anatomy may directly interfere with oocyte pick up, tubal transportation and fertilisation. However, in mild or minimal disease it might be the hostile peritoneal environment with increased macrophages, cytokines and vasoactive substances in the peritoneal fluid that is hampering fertility. Other potential factors include poor oocyte quality and dysfunction of fallopian tube and ovary. Though surgery helps to improve pregnancy rates in mild or minimal disease [10], assisted reproductive techniques continue to be the mainstay of treatment for endometriosis-associated infertility.

Signs suggestive of endometriosis may be noted during bimanual examination of the pelvis and include tethering of pelvic organs with restricted mobility of the uterus, palpable nodules or visible lesions of endometriosis in posterior fornix of vagina, and tenderness. However, signs may be subtle and a normal examination does not exclude endometriosis [9].

One of the key challenges in diagnosing endometriosis arises from a considerable overlap in symptoms of endometriosis with other conditions such as chronic pelvic inflammatory disease (PID), interstitial cystitis and irritable bowel syndrome (IBS). Diagnosis is suspected on the basis of clinical symptoms and confirmed by laparoscopy. A normal abdominal and pelvic examination, ultrasound and magnetic resonance imaging (MRI) do not necessarily exclude endometriosis. If

there is a high clinical suspicion based on symptoms further investigations should be considered [9].

Laparoscopy Direct visualisation of endometriotic lesions at laparoscopy (visual inspection of the abdominopelvic cavity) remains the gold standard for the diagnosis of the disease. Histological confirmation is recommended, though a negative result does not always reliably exclude endometriosis. Laparoscopy also allows evaluation of the stage and the site of the disease.

Transvaginal Ultrasound and MRI Diagnostic modalities such as transvaginal ultrasonography (TVS) and MRI perform poorly in the detection of peritoneal implants and adhesions. However, both have high sensitivity (80%–90%) and specificity (60%–98%) in detecting ovarian endometrioma. TVS is preferred over MRI as the primary investigation of choice in the diagnosis of endometrioma, owing to its low cost. Pelvic MRI should be considered to assess the extent of deep endometriosis involving the bowel, bladder or ureters to assist with plans for surgical treatment.

Biomarkers in Serum and Endometrial Tissue Serum levels of cancer antigen 125 (CA-1250) may be elevated in endometriosis, but this test is of limited value for diagnostic purposes because of poor sensitivity and specificity. There is limited evidence available regarding specificity and sensitivity of other serum biomarkers such as human epididymis protein 4 (HE-4) or endometrial biomarkers such as the nerve fibre marker protein gene product 9.5 (PGP 9.5). Routine use of biomarkers to diagnose or monitor endometriosis is not recommended.

Table 3.1 briefly summarises the symptoms, signs and investigations for endometriosis.

3.6 Socioeconomic Burden and Psychosocial Impact

The delay in diagnosis and chronic nature of symptoms [11] adversely affects the health of women with endometriosis. The Global Study of Women's Health (GSWH), a large cross-sectional study conducted across 16 hospitals in 10 countries, reported a significantly reduced health-related quality of life (HRQoL), affecting both the physical and mental health of women with endometriosis when compared to those with similar symptoms but no endometriosis. Presence of endometriosis was associated with

Table 3.1 Symptoms, signs and investigations for the diagnosis of endometriosis

Symptoms of endometriosis
Dysmenorrhoea (painful periods severe enough to affect daily activities or quality of life)
Deep dyspareunia (deep pain during or after intercourse)
Cyclical dyschezia (painful bowel movement during periods)
Cyclical dysuria or haematuria (pain when passing urine or blood in urine during periods)
Chronic pelvic pain
Infertility alone or in combination with any of the aforementioned symptoms
May be completely asymptomatic

Signs of endometriosis
No detectable signs in minimal or mild endometriosis
Reduced pelvic organ mobility, tender nodularity in pouch of Douglas, palpable adnexal masses, vaginal endometriotic nodules may be seen in moderate to severe endometriosis

Investigations
Transvaginal ultrasound
First line investigation in women presenting with infertility and pelvic pain
High specificity and sensitivity to detect ovarian endometrioma – ground-glass appearance
Ability to detect deep rectovaginal disease – training and expertise required
Unable to detect superficial peritoneal lesions
Magnetic resonance imaging
Generally reserved for women where moderate to severe endometriosis with deep disease or rectovaginal/ureteric involvement is suspected
High specificity and sensitivity to detect deep endometriotic implants and ovarian endometrioma
Unable to detect superficial endometriotic lesions
Laparoscopy
Gold standard for diagnosis of endometriosis by visualisation of lesions
Histologic confirmation desirable but not essential
Allows evaluation of extent of lesions, site and stage of endometriosis
Ablation and excision of minimal, mild and up to moderate endometriosis is done at the same time as diagnostic laparoscopy for treatment of pain and/or infertility

a significant increase in time off work, with an average work productivity loss of 10.8 hours per week [11]. The economic burden (direct and indirect costs) associated with endometriosis is comparable to that of other chronic diseases (e.g. diabetes, Crohn's disease, rheumatoid arthritis). The indirect costs attributed to the loss of productivity was twice compared to the direct health care costs (physician visits, investigations, hospitalisation and surgery) [12].

Women with endometriosis suffer a higher dysfunction for social adjustment, have higher anxiety scores and more psychotic problems compared to those with non-endometriotic pelvic pain. The chronic recurrent pain of endometriosis can be debilitating, leading to fatigue, depression and insomnia. Deep dyspareunia, a common symptom of endometriosis, adversely impacts relationships and can negatively affect a woman's self-esteem and image.

3.7 Management of Endometriosis

Women with endometriosis may experience infertility, pain or both.

3.7.1 Management of Infertility Associated with Endometriosis

Women with endometriosis and subfertility should be referred to a specialist clinic for a complete fertility assessment of the couple.

Hormonal Treatment Hormonal agents that lead to ovarian suppression (e.g. gonadotropin-releasing hormone analogues [GnRHa], combined oral contraceptive pill [COCP] or Danazol), which are used for treatment of endometriosis associated pain, are not recommended, as they have not been found to be effective for treatment of infertility.

Surgery In women with minimal to mild endometriosis laparoscopic treatment (ablation, excision or adhesiolysis) has been shown to improve spontaneous pregnancy rates, though comparative effectiveness of various surgical techniques is less well known. The evidence is less robust with regards to moderate to severe endometriosis. Data from prospective cohort studies have shown that laparoscopic treatment to moderate to severe disease is associated with a higher pregnancy rate (52%–69%) compared to expectant management (0%–30%).

In women with ovarian endometrioma, cystectomy with stripping of capsule compared to drainage and fulguration of endometrioma is associated with a higher postoperative spontaneous pregnancy rate. Both techniques can potentially compromise ovarian reserve. Surgery for deep endometriosis and rectovaginal disease is complex and carries high morbidity. Surgery for the sole purpose of improving fertility is rarely used and more often done for associated pain. A shared decision-making process should take into account co-existing pain, chances of spontaneous conception, access to assisted reproduction and risks of surgery.

Medically Assisted Reproduction Medically assisted reproduction is widely used for the treatment of endometriosis associated infertility. In women with minimal to mild endometriosis, controlled ovarian simulation with gonadotropins and intrauterine insemination (IUI) is more effective than both expectant management and IUI alone in increasing rates of live birth rate and pregnancy rate respectively. In vitro fertilisation (IVF) is the treatment of choice in women with moderate and severe endometriosis, where other treatments have failed or where there is associated tubal or male factor infertility. Data from systematic reviews have shown that following IVF, women with stage I and II endometriosis have implantation, clinical pregnancy and live birth rates similar to those of women with other causes of infertility. Presence of stage III and IV endometriosis was associated with a lower implantation and clinical pregnancy rate with a trend towards reduction in the live birth rate, though the latter did not reach clinical significance. A limited number of studies of variable quality have shown that treatment with GnRHa for 3–6 months prior to IVF improves clinical pregnancy rates.

In women with unilateral endometrioma seeking IVF, preoperative ovarian cystectomy does not improve cycle outcome. Decision to operate in such cases should be balanced against the risks of surgery including the loss of ovarian reserve and management of associated pain.

3.7.2 Management of Pain Associated with Endometriosis

Various hormonal medications and analgesics are used in women with suspected endometriosis, even before the diagnosis is confirmed by laparoscopy.

Pharmacological Treatment Endometriosis is an oestrogen dependent condition. Ovarian suppression with hormones is used to control symptoms of endometriosis. They have an added advantage of reducing heavy menstrual bleeding, a common symptom of adenomyosis that often coexists with endometriosis.

Hormonal treatments commonly used are combined oral contraceptives, progestogens (e.g. Depo Provera injections, progestogen only pills, levo-norgesterel intra-uterine system, gestrinone), antiprogestogens, aromatase inhibitors and gonadotropin releasing hormone agonists (GnRHa) combined with steroidal and non-steroidal analgesics. The evidence related to neuromodulators is insufficient. There is no concrete evidence available to support one treatment choice over another – the treatment options are individualised and often discretionary following an informed discussion with the woman [2]. Both progestogens and the combined oral contraceptive pill are the first-line hormonal treatment for endometriosis and may be initiated in primary care in women with symptoms suspected of endometriosis. Medical treatment provides transient symptom relief with resurgence of symptoms once medications are stopped and hormonal treatment is not compatible with attempts to become pregnant.

Surgery Surgery remains the mainstay in the diagnosis and treatment of endometriosis and the preferred treatment choice for women trying to conceive, as hormonal medications interfere with conception. With advances in laparoscopic surgery a 'see and treat' policy is often employed for minimal, mild and up to moderate endometriosis. Endometriotic lesions are either excised or ablated at the time of initial diagnostic laparoscopy. Recurrence of symptoms is common after treatment, with reported rates of 30%–50% at 5 years [13]. Given the paucity of effective medical treatment and high recurrence rates, women with endometriosis often undergo multiple operations in an attempt to alleviate their symptoms. Removal of the ovaries is associated with the least risk of recurrence and is often combined with hysterectomy in those who have concomitant menstrual problems or adenomyosis. Oophorectomy with or without hysterectomy is used as a last resort when all other alternatives have failed and fertility is no longer a priority.

3.8 Organisation of Care

Women with endometriosis are looked after in primary, secondary and tertiary care settings [9]. Following an initial assessment in primary care, women with suspected endometriosis are offered an empirical trial of hormonal treatment in the form of progestogens or the combined oral contraceptive pill with analgesics. In those whose symptoms persist, are unable to tolerate hormones or wish fertility, referral to secondary care should be made for further investigations and consideration of laparoscopy. At laparoscopy minimal and mild disease is usually treated by ablation or excision. Those with moderate to severe disease involving, bowel, ureter or bladder are referred to tertiary endometriosis centres with access to advanced laparoscopic surgeons, colorectal surgeons, urologists, pain specialists and specialist nurses.

Conclusion

Endometriosis associated infertility presents a particular challenge for patients and clinician who need to balance the need to facilitate conception alongside the need to control symptoms of pain. Cases are best managed in a multidisciplinary setting with specialist input form endometriosis surgeons and assisted reproduction specialists.

References

1. Burney RO, Giudice LC., Pathogenesis and pathophysiology of endometriosis. *Fertil Steril* 2012;**98** (3):511–19.

2. Dunselman GA, Vermeulen N, Becker C, et al. and European Society of Human Reproduction and Embryology. ESHRE guideline: Management of women with endometriosis. *Hum Reprod (Oxf)*, 2014;**29**(3): 400–12.

3. Gruppo italiano per lo studio dell'endometriosi. Prevalence and anatomical distribution of endometriosis in women with selected gynaecological conditions: results from a multicentric Italian study. Gruppo italiano per lo studio dell'endometriosi. *Hum Reprod (Oxf)* 1994;**9**(6):1158–62.

4. American Society for Reproductive Medicine. Revised American Society for Reproductive Medicine classification of endometriosis: 1996. *Fertil Steril.* 1997;**67**(5):817–21.

5. Bricou A, Batt RE, Chapron C. Peritoneal fluid flow influences anatomical distribution of endometriotic lesions: Why Sampson seems to be right. *Eur J Obstet Gynecol Reprod Biol* 2008; **138**(2):127–34.

6. Cramer DW, Missmer SA. The epidemiology of endometriosis. *Ann NY Acad Sci* 2002;**955**:11–22; discussion 34–6, 396–406.

7. Bravi F, Parazzini F, Cipriani S, Chiaffarino F, Ricci E, Chiantera V, Vigano P, La Vecchia C., Tobacco smoking and risk of endometriosis: a systematic review and meta-analysis. *BMJ Open* 2014;**4**(12): e006325-2014–006325.

8. Parazzini F, Cipriani S, Bravi F, Pelucchi C, Chiaffarino F, Ricci E, Vigano P. A metaanalysis on alcohol consumption and risk of endometriosis. *Am J Obstet Gynecol* 2013;**209** (2):106.e1–106.10.

9. NICE (National Institute of Care and Excellence). Endometriosis: Diagnosis and management. NICE guideline NG73, September 2017.

10. Duffy JM, Arambage K, Correa FJ., et al. Laparoscopic surgery for endometriosis. *Cochrane Database Syst Rev* 2014;(**4**):CD011031.

11. Nnoaham KE, Hummelshoj L, Webster P, et al. and World Endometriosis Research Foundation Global Study of Women's Health, Consortium. Impact of endometriosis on quality of life and work productivity: A multicenter study across ten countries. *Fertil Steril* 2011;**96** (2):366–73.e8.

12. Simoens S, Dunselman G, Dirksen C, et al. The burden of endometriosis: Costs and quality of life of women with endometriosis and treated in referral centres. *Hum Reprod (Oxf)* 2012;**27**(5):1292–9.

13. Guo SW., Recurrence of endometriosis and its control. *Hum Reprod Update* 2009;**15**(4):441–61.

Uterine and Tubal Causes of Infertility

Abha Maheshwari

4.1 Background

Tubal abnormalities alone or in combination with other factors account for 17%–25% of all couples who present with infertility. Their prevalence is higher in older women and those with secondary infertility [1].

Restriction of tubal function due to pelvic adhesions or tubal damage (in the form of occlusion or fibrosis) results in impairment of the ability of the fallopian tube to effectively transport an egg or embryo to the uterus. The amount of damage can vary greatly in extent, anatomical location and nature. Tubal disease can involve the proximal, distal or entire tube and varies in severity.

Abnormalities of uterine anatomy or function are relatively uncommon causes of infertility but should be considered through appropriate history and investigation.

4.2 Causes of Tubal Factor Infertility

There are multiple conditions associated with uterine and tubal factor infertility (Table 4.1). Pelvic inflammatory disease (PID) is the most common cause of tubal disease, representing more than 50% of cases, and may affect the fallopian tube at multiple sites. The most common infective agent involved is *Chlamydia trachomatis*. The risk of acquiring chlamydial infection is increased through multiple sexual partners.

Previous extensive pelvic surgery can lead to altered anatomy and the formation of tubal adhesions leading to tubal blockage. Appendicitis leading to peritonitis is a classic example where significant adhesions may form involving the fallopian tubes. Even if the adhesions formed appear to involve only one tube, it is possible that the contralateral tube although macroscopically normal may be compromised. This is similar to the situation which might arise following an ectopic pregnancy.

One of the challenges facing clinicians is the fact that following elaborate investigations (including

Table 4.1 Factors associated with tubal and uterine anomalies

Tubal	Uterine
Pelvic inflammatory disease	Adenomyosis
Past *Chlamydia* infection	Uterine septum
Multiple sexual partners	Polyps
Previous pelvic surgery	Fibroids
Previous ruptured appendix	Intrauterine adhesions
History of inflammatory	(Asherman's
bowel disease	syndrome)
Previous ectopic pregnancy	Mullerian anomalies
Endometriosis	

tubal assessment), it is often difficult to provide infertile couples with an accurate prognosis. For women with infertility due to tubal disease, predicting the chance of pregnancy with or without corrective surgery often remains imprecise. There is no universally accepted classification of tubal disease severity to provide comparability of published results. It is acknowledged that the chances of conception are low in women with bilateral tubal occlusion and good in women with patent tubes with few filmy adhesions. The Hull & Rutherford classification [2] is a simple classification system that separates infertile women into three categories according to the severity of tubal damage (Table 4.2).

Other classification systems have been designed including those from the American Fertility Society [3], Akande [4] and others. Although, such systems are descriptive of the extent of disease, there remains a lack of robust data to correlate with prognosis.

4.3 Other Pelvic Pathology

4.3.1 Fibroids

Uterine leiomyomas, commonly called fibroids, occur, to varying degree, in as many as 20% of women of reproductive age. Fibroids are benign tumours of smooth muscle growing within the uterus.

Table 4.2 'H and R' classification

Class	Name	Description
1	Minor/grade I	Tubal fibrosis absent even if tube occluded (proximally) Tubal distension absent even if tube occluded (distally) Mucosal appearances favourable Adhesions (peri tubal-ovarian) are flimsy
2	Intermediate or moderate/grade II	Unilateral severe tubal damage, with or without contralateral minor disease 'Limited' dense adhesions of tubes and/or ovaries
3	Severe/grade III	Bilateral tubal damage, tubal fibrosis, extensive tubal distension >1.5 cm, Abnormal mucosal appearance, bilateral occlusion, 'extensive' dense adhesions

Source: Ref. [2].

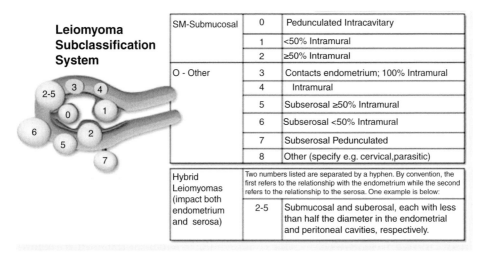

Leiomyoma Subclassification System			
SM-Submucosal	0	Pedunculated Intracavitary
	1	<50% Intramural
	2	≥50% Intramural
O - Other	3	Contacts endometrium; 100% Intramural
	4	Intramural
	5	Subserosal ≥50% Intramural
	6	Subserosal <50% Intramural
	7	Subserosal Pedunculated
	8	Other (specify e.g. cervical, parasitic)
Hybrid Leiomyomas (impact both endometrium and serosa)		Two numbers listed are separated by a hyphen. By convention, the first refers to the relationship with the endometrium while the second refers to the relationship to the serosa. One example is below:
	2-5	Submucosal and suberosal, each with less than half the diameter in the endometrial and peritoneal cavities, respectively.

Figure 4.1 Classification of fibroids.
Adapted from Munro MG, Critchley HO, Broder MS, Fraser IS; for the FIGO Working Group on Menstrual Disorders.
FIGO classification system (PALM-COEIN) for causes of abnormal uterine bleeding in non-gravid women of reproductive age.
Int J Gynecol Obstet. 2011;113:3–13 [5]

Malignant transformation is very rare. Various classification systems of fibroids exist usually based on the location of the tumour within the uterus (submucosal, intramural and subserosal). Further subdivisions based on the proportion of the fibroid within the uterine muscle wall at each location are shown in Figure 4.1 and used by most societies and research trials.

How much impact fibroids have on fertility has been a matter of debate. It is unclear as to whether the finding of fibroids in infertile women is incidental or causative. In addition, there is controversy as to whether the association applies only to the chances of spontaneous conception or has a bearing on the outcome of fertility treatment. Some of the reasons for controversy within the literature relate to the variety of types of fibroids, inconsistency of the nomenclature used, heterogeneity in study design and a lack of appropriately powered randomised trials. Despite these concerns it is accepted that fibroids are associated with infertility. Various causes have been postulated for this (Table 4.3). It is most probably a combination of factors that contributes to any associated fertility difficulties. However, the literature is inconsistent in assessing the impact that such disturbances might have on the likelihood of achieving and

Table 4.3 Mechanisms by which fibroids may impair fertility

Deformity of the cavity may affect implantation

Mechanical obstruction of the ostia of fallopian tubes

Chronic inflammatory response within the endometrium

Disordered uterine contractility associated with intramural fibroids

Endometrial atrophy due to pressure from a fibroid mass

maintaining pregnancy (with or without fertility treatment).

4.3.2 Endometriosis

Endometriosis encompasses a spectrum of disease ranging from minimal to severe. Many women with minimal and mild endometriosis experience no difficulty in conceiving. It is not unusual for parous women undergoing sterilisation to be noted to have endometriosis. However, it appears that the prevalence of endometriosis is higher in women attending fertility clinics compared to that in the general population, with some studies quoting up to 50%.

There is dispute over whether minimal/mild endometriosis is a causal finding in couples with infertility and whether or not treatment of this degree of endometriosis is of benefit. Moderate or severe endometriosis involving adhesions or ovarian cysts may impair fertility by inhibiting ovulation and/or ovum 'pick-up' by the Fallopian tubes. However, in studies involving infertile couples, the finding of minimal and mild endometriosis seems to be an added negative fertility factor. The exact mechanism of this negative fertility factor is unclear but various possible mechanisms have been postulated. Endometriosis as an issue in infertility is explored in more detail in Chapter 3.

4.3.3 Adenomyosis

Although often discovered in parous women, adenomyosis has been found to be associated with infertility. This is mainly due to effects on implantation. It is estimated that one third of all cases of endometriosis are associated with adenomyosis. However, studies on adenomyosis are limited in infertility populations and are frequently confounded by the presence of other factors. In the absence of agreed diagnostic criteria and the failure of national registries to consistently include the diagnosis, the exact prevalence and strength of the association of adenomyosis with infertility are not known.

4.3.4 Endometrial Polyps

It is estimated that uterine polyps are found in 10% of the general female population. Endometrial polyps are frequently seen in subfertile women, and there is some evidence suggesting a detrimental effect on fertility. How polyps contribute to subfertility and pregnancy loss is uncertain and possible mechanisms are poorly understood. It may be related to mechanical interference with sperm transport, embryo implantation or through intrauterine inflammation or altered production of endometrial receptivity factors.

4.3.5 Structural Uterine Abnormalities

Structural uterine anomalies are usually derived from deviation in development of mullerian or paramesonephric ducts. Abnormalities of uterine anatomy are relatively uncommon causes of infertility in women. Their effect on reproduction depend on type and degree. An internationally accepted classification has been produced by joint consensus between the European Society of Human Reproduction and Embryology (ESHRE) and the European Society of Gynaecological Endoscopy (ESGE) [6]. Anomalies are classified into main classes (Figure 4.2) expressing uterine anatomical deviations deriving from the same embryological origin. These are subdivided into subclasses expressing anatomical varieties with clinical significance. Cervical and vaginal anomalies are classified independently into subclasses having clinical significance.

It is difficult to ascertain whether such anomalies cause, or are just associated, with infertility given that there are often other factors associated with the infertility along with these findings. The location and degree of abnormality are also variable. Irrespective of this uncertainty, it is important to identify if these abnormalities are present, as they have implications for obstetric care as well as some aspects of fertility treatments. Mullerian anomalies are associated in a third of cases with renal and spinal cord abnormalities, the absence of one kidney being the most common abnormality.

4.3.6 Intrauterine Adhesions

The presence of adhesions within the uterine cavity may have profound effects on reproductive potential. The term Asherman's syndrome (AS) describes the clinical situation of absent or light periods, sometimes associated with pain and an inability to conceive consequent

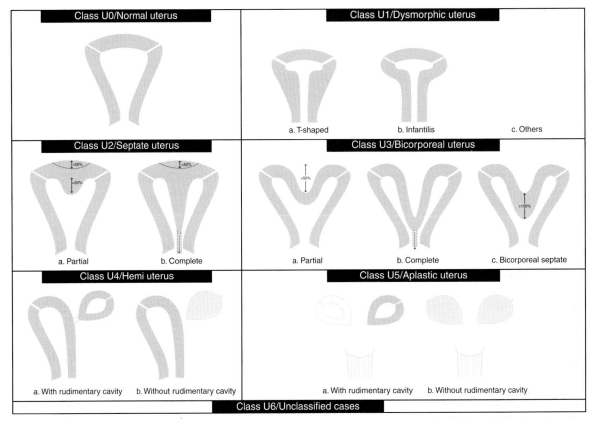

Figure 4.2 ESHRE/ESGE classification of uterine anomalies.
Reproduced from [6].

on damage to the endometrial cavity usually following curettage. AS causes infertility by reducing implantation potential.

While the degree of severity of intrauterine adhesions may be assessed by hysterosalpingography, in more recent years classifications systems have been developed based on hysteroscopy, now the gold standard to diagnose AS. The widely used AFS system includes an assessment of the extent of the disease, menstrual pattern and the density of the adhesions. Both hysteroscopy and hysterosalpingography could be used for this kind of scoring system (Figure 4.3).

4.4 Diagnosis

4.4.1 History Taking

A good structured history from the female partner is essential in evaluating the risk of uterine and tubal factors. A history of ectopic pregnancy, pelvic inflammatory disease (PID), endometriosis or prior pelvic surgery raises the index of suspicion for tubal factor infertility.

All patients in the fertility clinic should be asked these specific questions (Table 4.4). If endometriosis is suspected, it is essential to explore a history of dyspareunia, pain or difficulty at defaecation (dyschezia), or bleeding per rectum. These symptoms will assist in determining the potential extent of pathology as well as direct appropriate investigations. The impact symptoms have on quality of life should be evaluated at the initial consultation as that will influence decision making as to whether to treat pathology or proceed with fertility treatment.

4.4.2 Investigations

Investigations to diagnose uterine and tubal factor range from blood tests, radiological investigations to endoscopic evaluation. We will discuss each of the investigations, where they can be used and their limitations.

4.4.2.1 Chlamydia Antibody Testing

The detection of antibodies to *Chlamydia trachomatis* has been associated with tubal pathology: however, this test has limited clinical utility on its own. Compared with laparoscopy, the Chlamydia antibody test (CAT) has modest sensitivity (40%–50%) and positive predictive value (PPV) of 60%, but high negative predictive value (NPV) of 80%–90% for detection of distal tubal disease. PPV is the probability that subjects with a positive screening test truly have the disease (i.e. CAT positive has tubal disease). NPV is the probability that subjects with a negative screening test (CAT negative) truly do not have tubal disease. For patients with no risk factor a negative CAT indicates that there is less than a 15% chance of tubal pathology. CAT does not differentiate between remote and persistent infection, nor does it advise on actual tubal damage.

4.4.2.2 Two-Dimensional Ultrasound

A systematically conducted two-dimensional (2-D) ultrasound is a key initial tool for uterine and tubal evaluation. It is non-invasive, simple, low cost and available in almost every setting. All gynaecologists are familiar with the technique. Both transabdominal as well as transvaginal scans can provide useful information.

Table 4.4 Features in history suggestive of uterine/tubal factors

History of	Think of
• Multiple sexual partners • Previous pelvic inflammatory disease/ Chlamydia • Previous pelvic surgery • Ruptured appendix • History of colitis/ Crohn's disease	Tubal factors
• Heavy painful periods • Intermenstrual bleeding • Pressure symptoms • Previous uterine curettage • Recurrent miscarriage	Fibroids/endometriosis/ adenomyosis Asherman's syndrome Uterine anomalies
• Bleeding per rectum • Dyspareunia/dyschezia • Chronic pelvic pain	Endometriosis

The American Fertility Society's (AFS) classification of intrauterine adhesions

Look at...	Size/description	Score
Extent of cavity involved	<1/3	1
	1/3–2/3	2
	>2/3	4
Type of adhesions	Filmy	1
	Filmy and dense	2
	Dense	4
Menstrual pattern	Normal	0
	Hypomenorrhoea	2
	Amenorrhoea	4

Diagnostic table

Prognostic classification		HSG*	Hysteroscopy score
Stage I (mild)	1–4	....	....
Stage II (moderate)	5–8	....	....
Stage III (severe)	9–12	....	....
* All adhesions should be considered dense Additional findings..................			

Figure 4.3 Classification of Asherman's syndrome. Source: Ref. [3].

A basic 2-D US for evaluation of women from an infertility clinic should have minimum reporting criteria consisting of

- Day of cycle
- Endometrial thickness, irregularity/pattern
- Presence/absence of fibroids including number and location
- Presence of scar defect (in cases with previous caesarean section)
- Any features suggestive of adenomyosis
- Vaginal access to ovaries
- Antral follicle count
- Presence/absence of a pelvic cyst and its nature, that is, solid areas, complexity, thickness of wall, echogenicity (if present)
- Any other adnexal mass
- Pain during scan

A well conducted 2-D scan with a high index of suspicion for uterine and tubal factors has the potential to provide important information. For certain conditions, it may have to be done in a specific part of menstrual cycle; for example, in the early proliferative phase, when the endometrium is thin, it is easier to visualise intrauterine polyps.

Endometriomas are present in 17%–44% cases of endometriosis and these have a classic ground-glass appearance on 2-D ultrasound (Figure 4.4).

4.4.2.3 Role of Three-Dimensional Ultrasound

Although not freely available, most new machines now include this feature. Patients find 3-D vaginal ultrasound scans acceptable, there being no real difference from conventional ultrasound. Its reliability

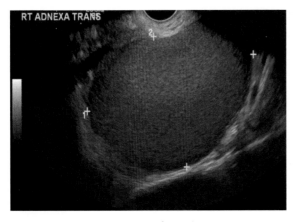

Figure 4.4 2-D ultrasound image of an endometrioma.

has been quoted as similar to that of MRI, especially for uterine lesions and anomalies. This is because imaging of the uterus can be presented in the sagittal, transverse and coronal planes in an objective way. It provides precise and objective measurements of the uterine dimensions, which is the absolute advantage in accurate assessment of uterine anomalies. However, its role in routine practice for every patient's evaluation is not proven. There are expenses associated with it in terms of the cost of equipment. Artefacts related to inappropriate volume acquisition could be an issue with 3-D ultrasound (3-D US) and so training of staff in image acquisition and post-processing techniques is important.

The role of 3-D US as a routine screening test has not been appropriately evaluated in the fertility clinic setting. Two-dimensional ultrasound (2-D US) is recommended for the evaluation of asymptomatic women. 3-D US is recommended for the diagnosis of female genital anomalies in 'symptomatic' patients belonging to high-risk groups for the presence of a female genital anomaly and in any asymptomatic woman suspected to have an anomaly from routine evaluation, for example, in cases of recurrent miscarriage.

As shown in Figure 4.5 an endometrial polyp in a well conducted 2-D US may be suspected, however, more detailed imaging is achievable with 3-D US.

For uterine anomalies, while 2-D US may raise suspicions of a problem, 3-D US provides more reliable information. This is illustrated in Figure 4.6, where it is shown that an appropriately acquired 3D image can delineate between various kinds of uterine anomalies by measuring uterine wall thickness and midline indentation.

4.4.2.4 Hysterosalpingography

Hysterosalpingography (**HSG**) has been a traditional first-line investigation for tubal patency. It has been widely available and offers printable films that could be re-evaluated at any time. It is based on injecting an oil soluble contrast media through the cervical canal and taking images under fluoroscopic guidance. In addition to tubal patency it offers additional useful information in cases of infertile women for potential intra-cavitary pathology (presence of defects). There may also be a therapeutic role in tubal flushing (see Chapter 6), with a number of small randomised trials suggesting improved pregnancy rates. It does involve exposure to radiation and for this reason a number of clinics are now moving on to a newer method of tubal evaluation called hysterosalpingo-contrast sonography (HyCoSy).

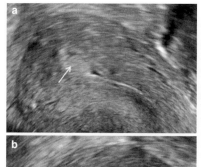

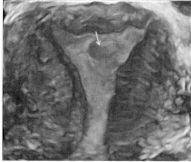

Figure 4.5 Comparison of 2-D and 3-D ultrasound for endometrial polyp. Reproduced from Ref. [7].

4.4.2.5 Hysterosalpingo-Contrast Sonography

HyCoSy is an ultrasound-based test of tubal patency. It involves a similar procedure to HSG, except that the flow of fluid instilled through the cervix into the uterine cavity and fallopian tubes is visualised using ultrasound rather than fluoroscopy. HyCoSy also provides additional information about uterine cavity lesions such as polyps/submucosa fibroids and so forth. It is minimally invasive, simple, low cost and potentially available in almost every clinic setting, as no radiological input is required. It has the advantage of being performed within the office setting and entails no exposure to radiation. Results are immediately available, enabling prompt decision making on further management.

Some specialists recommend that ultrasound-based assessment should be the first line investigation for tubal patency and that HSG should be abandoned where HyCoSy is available.

4.4.2.6 Diagnostic Laparoscopy

Diagnostic laparoscopy, while invasive and more costly, is the gold standard for diagnosing extra-cavitary uterine pathology, tubal and peritoneal factors. Surgical evaluation of the pelvis facilitates a 'see and treat' approach to simple pathology such as minimal/mild endometriosis and filmy tubal adhesions. The association of tubal factors with infertility could be due to obstruction and/or non-occlusive tubal damage. While HSG and HyCoSy can identify tubal blockage and patency, only laparoscopy will definitively identify the cases of non-

occlusive tubal damage, for example, tortuous, dilated tubes. One also has to remember that the identification of tubal patency alone does not guarantee normal tubal function.

4.4.2.7 Combined Laparoscopy and Hysteroscopy

This is usually needed to fully evaluate uterine anomalies. However, with better MRI and the increased utilisation of 3-D US, this is less frequently employed. If laparoscopy is needed for other reasons a combined hysteroscopy and laparoscopy approach may be useful.

4.4.2.8 Hysteroscopy

Hysteroscopy is used to diagnose and treat uterine lesions such as polyps/fibroids/uterine septum/intra-uterine adhesions and so forth. There is no evidence that routine hysteroscopy improves the outcome of fertility treatments and thus it should be performed only for a definite indication. More and more clinics are now performing out-patient procedures, and the indications for in-patient hysteroscopy under general anaesthesia in this group are diminishing.

4.4.2.9 Magnetic Resonance Imaging

MRI is non-invasive and involves no exposure to radiation. It gives a reliable and objective representation of the examined organs in three dimensions. It is particularly useful in assessing the extent of endometriosis, diagnosing adenomyosis, confirming the number and position of fibroids as well as in the evaluation of uterine anomalies.

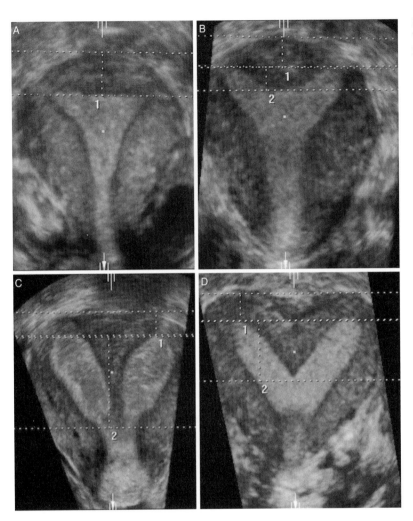

Figure 4.6 3-D ultrasound for delineating the uterine anomalies.
Source: Ref. [6].

4.4.2.10   A Pathway of Pelvic Evaluation

In evaluating pelvic anatomy a careful history and the use of 2-D US should enable identification of at risk patients and direct further workup (Figure 4.7).

4.5   Treatments

Treatment for uterine and tubal factor infertility depends on the condition identified. There are only a few treatments with definite benefit, and in other situations multiple factors have to be taken into consideration.

4.5.1   Fibroids

There has been significant controversy whether removal of a leiomyoma improves fertility and pregnancy outcome. Most data evaluating the impact of fibroids on fertility are derived from observational studies. Definitive clinical recommendations are difficult to make due to study heterogeneity in relation to the location and size of leiomyomas, the variety of resulting clinical symptoms and the range of methodology and clinical end-points used in the available literature.

If fibroids are diagnosed an individualised assessment should be made based on the following:

- Fibroid factors
  - ○   Size, numbers, symptoms, previous surgery, associated pathology, and so forth
- Patient factors
  - ○   Age

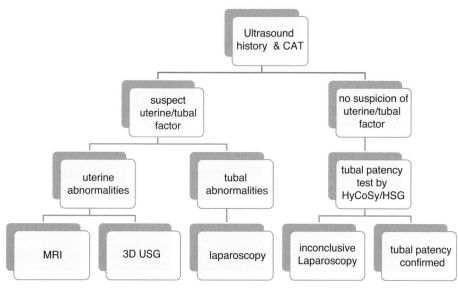

Figure 4.7 Suggested investigative pathway for uterine and tubal factor infertility.

- ○ History
- ○ Ovarian reserve
- ○ Type of treatment
- • Clinician factors
- ○ Expertise

Subserosal fibroids usually do not affect fertility, unless they are compressing on the fallopian tubes, and should be operated on only if vaginal access to the ovaries for the purposes of egg collection in IVF is impaired or if the bulk of the tumour causes significant pressure symptoms. There is controversy about the appropriate management of intramural fibroids. An individualised assessment based on the aforementioned factors in a multidisciplinary team setting involving the patient should be made. Hysteroscopic myomectomy for a cavity distorting leiomyoma improves clinical pregnancy rates but there is insufficient evidence regarding the impact of this procedure on likelihood of a live birth rate or a reduction in early pregnancy loss [8].

4.5.2 Tubal Surgery

With increased popularity and success of in vitro fertilisation, tubal surgery is being performed less frequently and available surgical expertise and experience is diminishing. Surgery entails operative risks (general anaesthetic, intraoperative and postoperative) and a high postoperative incidence of ectopic pregnancy. However, IVF is expensive and in some

areas of the United Kingdom is not publicly available in contrast to tubal surgery. Tubal surgery has the advantage of being a one-time intervention and does not require intense monitoring, as is the case in IVF. Many variables should be considered when counselling patients with tubal infertility regarding the choice between corrective surgery and IVF. These include the age of the woman, ovarian reserve, the number of children, the size and extent of tubal disease, the presence of other infertility factors, patient preference, religious beliefs and costs.

Surgery is considered a viable treatment option for women with mild tubal disease. Procedures such as salpingostomy (formation of an opening into a uterine tube for the purpose of drainage) or fimbrioplasty (breaking of scar tissue around the distal end of the tube) can be performed for distal tubal obstruction in young women with no other significant infertility factors. Reversal of sterilisation, if done at a younger age, may be more effective than IVF; however, this is not true for advanced reproductive age. There is evidence to recommend tubal cannulation for proximal tubal obstruction in young women with no other significant infertility factors. Laparoscopic salpingectomy before IVF has a role in improving livebirth rates among women with hydrosalpinges diagnosed on ultrasound [9].

Large trials with adequate power are warranted to establish the clinical and cost effectiveness of tubal surgery versus IVF in different age groups of women. Future trials should not only report livebirth rates per patient but should compare adverse effects and costs of treatment over a longer time.

> **Key Point**
>
> The ideal candidate for tubal surgery would be a young patient, with no other fertility factors present and where tubal blockage is amenable to surgery.

4.5.3 Endometriosis

Endometriosis in various stages is frequently found in the infertility population. There is evidence from randomised trials suggesting treatment of minimal and mild endometriosis leads to improvement in spontaneous pregnancy rates though these studies were carried out many years ago. No randomised controlled trial data on treatment of mild disease are available prior to assisted reproduction treatment.

Removal of endometriotic cysts has traditionally been recommended if found in women with subfertility. However, recent concerns have been raised about reduced ovarian reserve following surgery. There are no substantive data to suggest that operating on endometrioma improves live birth rates in IVF. However, almost all the available evidence is based on observational studies. Similarly, there is no evidence that operating on rectovaginal endometriosis improves the live birth rate prior to fertility treatment.

Randomised trials have suggested that, if operating on endometrioma, laparoscopic excision rather than drainage and ablation should be performed.

Any decision for surgery to endometriosis in women with subfertility should take in to consideration the age of the patient and other factors, for example, sperm quality, ovulatory dysfunction, the duration of infertility, existing ovarian reserve, ovarian access for IVF, the presence of symptoms affecting quality of life as well as patient choice. These decisions should ideally be determined in a multidisciplinary team discussion where the potential morbidity associated with surgery should also be considered.

4.5.4 Adenomyosis

Multiple techniques have been advocated for treatment of adenomyosis such as adenomyomectomy, high-intensity focused ultrasound, myomectomy, uterine artery embolization, hysterotomy, wedge resection and so forth [10]. However, there are no good quality data to provide certainty that any improves the pregnancy rates either for spontaneous conception or following fertility treatment.

4.5.5 Endometrial Polyps

Endometrial polyps can be removed as part of a hysteroscopic procedure. Their removal in subfertile women is commonly performed with an aim to improve reproductive outcome. However, the evidence suggesting clinical benefit with this approach prior to assisted reproduction technology is weak. Currently, there are insufficient data to recommend routine surgical removal of an endometrial polyp, especially when identified for the first time during ovarian stimulation for in vitro fertilisation.

To date, the available low-quality evidence suggests that hysteroscopic removal of endometrial polyps suspected on ultrasound in women prior to intrauterine insemination (IUI) may improve the clinical pregnancy rate compared to simple diagnostic hysteroscopy. This is based on the data from one randomised trial where women underwent either hysteroscopic removal of polyps or diagnostic hysteroscopy only. A recent Cochrane review suggests that further research is needed to determine the clinical benefit, if any, of the hysteroscopic treatment of suspected major uterine cavity abnormalities in women with unexplained subfertility or prior to IUI, IVF or intra-cytoplasmic sperm injection (ICSI).

4.5.6 Intrauterine Adhesions

The treatment strategy for Asherman's syndrome can be summarised in four main steps:

- Treatment (dilatation and curettage, hysteroscopy, hysterotomy)
- Re-adhesion prevention (intrauterine device, uterine balloon stent, Foley's catheter, anti-adhesion barriers)
- Restoring normal endometrium (hormonal treatment, stem cells)
- Post-operative assessment (repeat surgery; diagnostic hysteroscopy; ultrasound).

These cases are few in number and sometimes several surgical procedures, over a period of some months, are needed to achieve an optimal outcome. It is important that women are counselled about this and the fact that despite surgery the overall prognosis for the development of normal endometrium and restoration of fertility remains poor.

4.5.7 Uterine Anomalies

Treatment of uterine anomalies depend on the type.

Arcuate Uterus No treatment is required, as the finding is not thought to impact on the chance of spontaneous conception or treatment-related fertility.

Septate Uterus Treatment is indicated only if there is a history of recurrent miscarriage. For those in whom there is no history of miscarriage but there is a history of infertility, treatment should be started only after counselling of uncertain benefit. While the uterine cavity would be expected to have healed within 2 months of surgery, there is insufficient evidence to advocate a specific length of time before a woman should conceive.

Bicornuate Uterus This has implications for obstetrics outcome, but no treatment is indicated in infertility, as there is no evidence that intervention improves the outcome either for spontaneous conception or following fertility treatment.

Key Points

There is good evidence that removal of hydrosalpinx (diagnosed on ultrasound) improves live birth rate in IVF.

There is controversy about treatment for endometriosis and adenomyosis to improve fertility.

Reports on success following tubal surgery are difficult to interpret and compare, due to imprecise terminology and differences in classification systems.

Submucosal fibroids affect embryo implantation rate in IVF; there is controversy about the impact of intramural fibroids; subserosal fibroids do not affect fertility.

4.6 Prevention

4.6.1 Tubal Factor Infertility

4.6.1.1 Primary Prevention

Health education about sexually transmitted disease is very important in order to reduce the risk of acquiring infection and the consequent hazard of tubal damage.

4.6.1.2 Secondary Prevention

Early diagnosis of sexually transmitted disease and contact tracing of those exposed will limit the risk of damage to the fallopian tubes.

4.6.2 Uterine Factor Infertility

Intrauterine adhesion formation could be minimised in the following circumstances:

- Hysteroscopic surgery
  - Careful surgical technique
  - Use of antiadhesive agents (though evidence is limited)
- Evacuation of retained products of conception
  - Surgical removal of retained products of conception in conditions such as incomplete or missed miscarriage should be performed with great care and, in favourable cases, a less invasive approach should be considered. Hysteroscopy, in experienced hands, can be an effective method for selective removal of placental retained tissue with good results in terms of pregnancy rates and prevention of intrauterine adhesions.

4.7 Conclusions

Uterine and tubal factors are associated with infertility. However, most of the conditions in this domain are linked with infertility by association (except bilateral tubal block) rather than through definitive evidence of causation. The strength of any association is not clear for most diagnoses. The impact of treatment in improving fertility has been poorly evaluated.

A high index of suspicion of tubal and uterine pathology may be informed by a detailed history supported by 2-D US. Targeted investigation should be made to confirm the diagnosis. Management should take into consideration the age of the woman, the duration of infertility, symptoms, other causes of infertility, surgical hazards, funding as well as the patient's wishes.

There are no clear management strategies, as individualised decisions have to be made. Health education and primary/secondary prevention will have an impact on minimising the risk of tubal factor infertility due to acquired infection.

References

1. Maheshwari A, Hamilton M, Bhattacharya S. Effect of female age on the diagnostic categories of infertility. *Hum Reprod*. 2008;23(3):538–42.

2. Rutherford AJ, Jenkins JM. Hull and Rutherford classification of infertility. *Hum Fertil (Camb)*. 2002;**5** (1 Suppl):S41–5.

3. The American Fertility Society classifications of adnexal adhesions, distal tubal occlusion, tubal occlusion secondary to tubal ligation, tubal pregnancies, mullerian anomalies and intrauterine adhesions. *Fertil Steril.* 1988;**49**:944–55.

4. Akande VA. Tubal disease: towards a classification. *Reprod BioMed.* 2007;**15**:369–75.

5. Munro MG, Critchley HO, Broder MS, Fraser IS for the FIGO Working Group on Menstrual Disorders. FIGO classification system (PALM-COEIN) for causes of abnormal uterine bleeding in nongravid women of reproductive age. *Int J Gynecol Obstet.*2011;**113**:3–13.

6. Grimbizis GF, Di Spiezio Sardo A, Saravelos SH, et al. The Thessaloniki ESHRE/ESGE consensus on diagnosis of female genital anomalies. *Hum Reprod.* 2016;**31**(1):2–7.

7. Chami A, Saridogan E. Endometrial polyps and subfertility. *J Obstet Gynaecol India.* 2017;**67**(1):9–14.

8. ASRM (Practice Committee of American Society of Reproductive Medicine). Removal of myoma in asymptomatic patients to improve fertility and/or reduce miscarriage rate: A guideline. *Fertil Steril.* 2017;**108**:416–25.

9. ASRM (Practice Committee of American Society of Reproductive Medicine). Role of tubal surgery in era of assisted reproductive technology: a committee opinion. *Fertil Steril.* 2015;**103**(6):e37–43. DOI: 10.1016/j.fertnstert.2015.03.032.

10. Maheshwari A, Gurunath S, Fatima F, Bhattacharya S. Adenomyosis and subfertility: a systematic review of prevalence, diagnosis, treatment and fertility outcomes. *Hum Reprod Update.* 2012;**18**(4):374–92.

Further Reading

Chua SJ, Akande VA, Mol BWJ. Surgery for tubal infertility. *Cochrane Database of Syst Rev* 2017; (1): CD006415. DOI: 10.1002/14651858.CD006415.pub3.

El-Toukhy T, Campo R, Khalaf Y, et al. Hysteroscopy in recurrent in-vitro fertilisation failure (TROPHY): a multicentre, randomised controlled trial. *Lancet.* 2016;**387** (10038):2614–21.

Jayaprakasan K, Polanski L, Sahu B, Thornton JG, Raine-Fenning N. Surgical intervention versus expectant management for endometrial polyps in subfertile women. *Cochrane Database Syst Rev.* 2014;(8): CD009592. DOI: 10.1002/14651858.CD009592 .pub2.

National Collaborating Centre for Women's and Children's Health. *Fertility: assessment and treatment for people with fertility problems*, 2nd ed. London: RCOG Publications; 2013.

Practice Committee of the American Society for Reproductive Medicine. Diagnostic evaluation of the infertile female: a committee opinion. *Fertil Steril.* 2015;**103**: e44–50.

Practice Committee of the American Society for Reproductive Medicine. Removal of myomas in asymptomatic patients to improve fertility and/or reduce miscarriage rate: a guideline. *Fertil Steril* 2017;**108**:416–25.

Practice Committee of the American Society for Reproductive Medicine. Uterine septum: a guideline. *Fertil Steril.* 2016;**106**:530–40.

Royal College of Obstetricians & Gynaecologists. Uterine and tubal factor subfertility. https://elearning.rcog.org.uk// uterine-and-tubal-factor-subfertility/uterine-and-tubal-factor-infertility

Saridogan E, Becker CM, Feki A, and Working group of ESGE, ESHRE, and WES. Recommendations for the surgical treatment of endometriosis. Part 1: Ovarian endometrioma. *Gynecol Surg.* 2017;**14**(1):27.

Toaff R, Ballas S. Traumatic hypomenorrhea-amenorrhea (Asherman's syndrome). *Fertil Steril.* 1978;**30**(4):379–87.

Chapter 5

Andrology and Infertility

Allan Pacey and Kevin McEleny

5.1 Introduction

Reproductive problems in the male are a significant cause of infertility in heterosexual couples. For the general gynaecologist, or specialist in reproductive medicine, this is an important part of their infertility practice, but one in which they may feel less confident or have had little or no formal training. Moreover, in addition to the infertility of heterosexual couples, an understanding of male fertility is important in its own right given that increasing number of single men or homosexual couples may present in the clinic either for their own reproductive needs, or to take part as donors in the family building for single women or same-sex (female) couples. It is, therefore, important that the gynaecologist or reproductive medicine specialist has a good understanding of issues in clinical and laboratory andrology as outlined in this chapter.

5.2 The Male Reproductive Tract and Physiology

A schematic diagram of the male reproductive tract is shown in Figure 5.1 with an overview of the main endocrine mechanisms controlling testicular function in Figure 5.2.

In most boys, sperm production begins early in puberty at around age 13.5 years and in most individuals continues relatively unhindered throughout life (but see Section 5.3). The starting point of spermatogenesis is a population of testicular stem cells in the germinal epithelium which begin to proliferate and self-renew, sending copies of themselves down a pathway of differentiation to make sperm. Most of the stages of spermatogenesis take place in a close connection with Sertoli cells over around 74 days (95% confidence interval [CI]: 69–80 days). Since each Sertoli cell can only support a finite number of developing sperm at any one time, the number of Sertoli cells (as evidenced by testicular volume) is the factor limiting how many sperm a testis can produce

per unit time. Spermatogenesis typically takes place in a 'wave-like' manner along the seminiferous tubule, suggesting some element of paracrine or autocrine coordination. The developing stages of sperm undergo meiotic divisions to generate sperm with half the number of chromosomes while at the same time, the sperm differentiate into the familiar plan of head, midpiece and tail (see Figure 5.3) as they pass through Sertoli cells and are released into the lumen.

Fully differentiated sperm released into the lumen of seminiferous tubules are not motile and are therefore moved gently by cilia, muscular contractions and back-pressure along to the efferent ducts and into the epididymis. Their passage along the epididymis typically takes about 7 to 10 days and it is during this time that sperm develop the capacity to become motile and also acquire the ability to bind to the egg. These functions are probably obtained through a series of modifications to surface proteins by epididymal secretions, although the exact details are not clear.

Compared to other mammals, there is limited sperm storage capacity within the human male reproductive tract to store sperm once they have finished epididymal maturation and before they are ejaculated. However, some sperm are probably stored in the cauda epididymis and testicular portion of the vas deferens. When ejaculation occurs, there is a 'pinching' of the muscular walls of the vas deferens and a bolus of sperm forced along it by peristaltic contractions towards the penile urethra. The process of ejaculation is highly coordinated and is normally associated with the release of a series of fluid 'fractions' in which sperm and fluid from the prostate tend to be in the first and second fractions and secretions from the seminal vesicles the later ones. This has implications for semen collection in diagnostic laboratories (where if the first fraction is not collected this can have an impact on the results of semen analysis) and for those couples practising 'coitus interruptus' as a form of contraception.

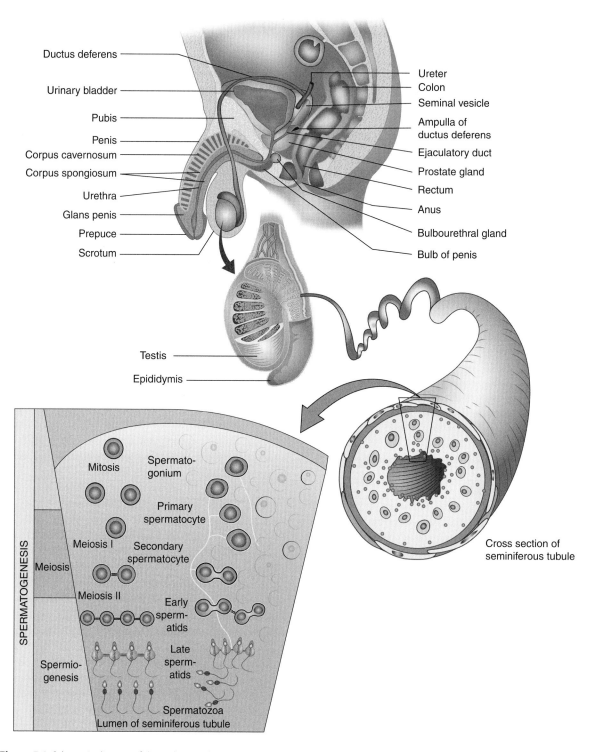

Figure 5.1 Schematic diagram of the male reproductive tract.

5.3 Causes of Male Subfertility

To determine the likely cause of male factor infertility, it is helpful for the clinician to place the patient into a mechanistic category. One approach is to divide the causes of male subfertility into (1) pre-testicular (those affecting the regulatory hormonal pathway); (2) testicular (those which relate to impaired testicular function); or (3) post-testicular (where there is a blockage of the male genital tract or other problems with associated ejaculation or sperm delivery). However, it is important to consider that there can be more than one cause.

5.3.1 Pre-testicular Causes

The development of the male urogenital system during neonatal life is under the primary control of the *SRY* gene. From about week 7 of gestation, this leads

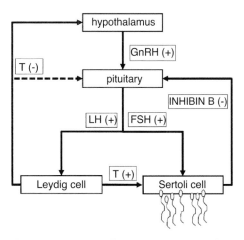

Figure 5.2 Overview of the endocrine control of testicular function.

to the development of the indifferent gonad to the male phenotype which can be clearly seen by about week 12. This is largely driven by a rise in fetal testosterone which triggers the regression of the mullerian duct system and the subsequent differentiation of the Wolffian ducts. A key part of the process is the trans-abdominal migration of the testis from the abdominal wall to the inner inguinal ring which occurs from weeks 10 to 23 of gestation. The failure to migrate correctly leads to cryptorchidism, with lifelong consequences for fertility. Also, during this time, fetal testosterone is thought to contribute to the proliferation of Sertoli cell numbers that directly influences the maximum sperm production in adulthood, as outlined earlier. It is suggested that the anogenital distance (the distance between the midpoint of the anus to the underside of the scrotum) in adults is a readout of androgen exposure in utero. However, while it broadly correlates with testis size, sperm production and fertility it is not sufficient to be diagnostic.

Less common are gene defects that affect the secretion of gonadotropin-releasing hormone (GnRH) from the hypothalamus, leading to congenital hypogonadotropic hypogonadism. The most common condition is Kallmann syndrome (affecting about 1 in 10,000 males) but there are many gene mutations which are thought to underpin this.

Finally, there are a number (acquired) of endocrine disorders that may lead to pre-testicular causes of male subfertility, including pituitary tumours (e.g. Cushing syndrome) or traumatic brain injury. Exogenous testosterone administered either medically as replacement therapy or by individuals in order to build muscle mass as part of sporting activity will cause a negative feedback on the hypothalamic–pituitary axis which in turn will reduce the secretion of luteinising hormone (LH) and follicle-stimulating

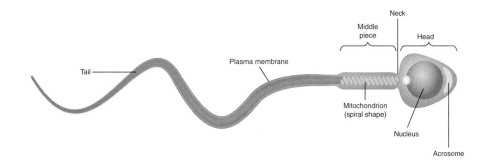

Figure 5.3 The ultrastructure of human spermatozoa.

hormone (FSH) which will lower (or abolish) sperm production (see Figure 5.2). While these effects can be reversed if the testosterone use is discontinued, this may take many months [1].

5.3.2 Testicular Causes

A number of genetic issues can trigger developmental problems which are associated with poor testicular development. These include Klinefelter's syndrome (typically 47 XXY but other variants are possible) which occurs in about 1 in 1,000 males. The testes in these men are typically small (<3.5 mL in volume) and histologically show degeneration of the seminiferous tubules, hyalinisation and fibrosis. Since the majority of genes which control spermatogenesis are located on the long arm of the Y chromosome, there are several key areas which are important for fertility. For example, men with (1) the AZFa microdeletion have Sertoli cell only syndrome; (2) the AZFb pattern have maturation arrest; and (3) AZFc have hypospermatogenesis.

One of the most common iatrogenic causes of testicular damage is as a consequence of chemotherapy or radiotherapy treatments delivered as part of cancer treatment. In each case, this can cause a depletion in the population of testicular stem cells which are the starting material for spermatogenesis (see Section 5.2). The extent of damage is difficult to predict in advance and seems to depend on the specific agents used as well as their dose and duration. Other prescription medicines can have similar effects although these are often poorly documented in the literature and so the clinician needs to be very thoughtful when taking a medical history.

Other testicular damage may be caused by varicoceles (an abnormal enlargement of the pampiniform venous plexus in the scrotum) and are more commonly seen in subfertile men. It is believed that they impair spermatogenesis through a heating effect, although the link between varicoceles and fertility is controversial. They can be observed during physical examination (see Section 5.4.1) and can be successfully treated by surgery (see Section 5.5.2).

Sexually transmitted infections (such as *Chlamydia trachomatis*) have the potential to influence male fertility as a consequence of the inflammatory reaction which may lead to tissue damage, the generation of free radicals from leucocytes or by direct damage on sperm by triggering apoptotic pathways [2]. The impact of other micro-organisms (e.g. *Neisseria gonorrhoea*/human papillomavirus) are less well understood, although have been implicated in poor reproductive outcome.

Some adult and post-pubertal infections such as mumps orchitis can dramatically influence testicular function, although historically has seen a decline in incidence due to childhood vaccination programmes. However, the controversy surrounding such vaccines in some parts of the world has led to a resurgence of cases. Damage is thought to occur because of direct damage to the germinal epithelium as well as by triggering an immunological reaction leading to the formation of sperm antibodies.

Lifestyle habits are a common concern for doctors and patients alike, often fuelled by media reports. Although there is some evidence that excessive alcohol intake, smoking of tobacco products (or cannabis), increases in testicular temperature due to occupation or choice of underwear [3] or some occupational chemical exposures (e.g. lead or glycol ether) can reduce semen quality, there is little evidence to date that lifestyle changes can improve matters and increase sperm quality or enhance fertility.

5.3.3 Post-testicular Causes

Post-testicular causes of male infertility relate to issues of sexual function, and male genital tract obstruction. The most common reason for azoospermia is vasectomy, but unintended vasal injury resulting in obstruction can occur as a consequence of groin surgery, such as hernia repair or orchidopexy. Non-iatrogenic causes include congenital absence of the vasa deferens, which is commonly linked to mutations in the cystic fibrosis (CF) genes. Obstruction can also be a consequence of genital tract infection. Whilst some of these causes may be suitable for genital tract reconstruction, many men will end up requiring surgical sperm retrieval for intra-cytoplasmic sperm injection (ICSI) (see Section 5.5.3).

Perhaps the most obvious reason for ejaculatory failure is in those men with spinal cord injury (SCI). In these men natural conception is rare because their ability to obtain a penile erection is usually impaired and as a consequence penile–vaginal intercourse is extremely difficult for them. Moreover, very few can achieve a normal (anterograde) ejaculation. Although sperm production is normally unaffected by their injury, because they ejaculate so infrequently, they often have samples with poor motility and an increased number of dead spermatozoa.

In some of men, anejaculation can be the reason for fertility problems and is usually due to peripheral nerve damage caused by generalised neuropathy (e.g. diabetes, or by damage to the pelvic plexi by surgery or trauma). Ejaculation requires intact sympathetic nerves (erections require parasympathetic pathways) and damage at any point from the relevant spinal cord segments to the genital tract can cause this problem.

In other men retrograde ejaculation can occur where at orgasm, sperm passes into the bladder due to bladder neck incompetence caused by surgery or drugs. Less commonly, ejaculatory duct obstruction caused by infection, cysts or calculi can result in anejaculation, often associated with pain at orgasm. In these men, semen follows the path of least resistance and sperm are deposited in the bladder (an obvious hindrance to fertility).

In men without any underlying physical or pharmacological cause, ejaculatory failure can still occur during intercourse and may have a psychosexual basis. It is important in such men therefore to enquire about libido and in their ability to reach orgasm. Anorgasmia and hypoactive sexual desire can have an endocrinological cause and those affected should be screened by checking their testosterone, prolactin and thyroid function (some clinicians also advocate checking oestrogen levels). Other causes can include medication, particularly drugs used to treat psychological disorders. However, disorders of libido and ejaculation are more commonly psychosexual in origin and may require referral for psychosexual counselling. Premature ejaculation is a common condition, but only rarely has an impact on fertility.

Erectile dysfunction (ED) becomes increasingly more common as men age, occurring in approximately 50% of men older than 50 years. Most ED is physical in origin and is related to the impact of the aging process on penile arteries and the corpora cavernosa. Problems are more commonly seen in men with diabetes, hypertension, cardiovascular disease and dyslipidaemia, so it is important that these parameters are checked when the patient reports an issue. Lifestyle factors such as obesity, cigarette smoking and excessive alcohol consumption are also relevant and should be enquired about. Hormonal factors such as a low testosterone or an elevated prolactin can be relevant also. ED is more common in subfertile men and may reflect an increased frequency or adverse health factors and psychological stress. The latter is more commonly seen in younger men, where it presents often suddenly with intermittent erections and the preservation of morning erections. ED of physical origins conversely is progressive, consistent and the patient will only rarely experience morning erections.

5.4 Investigation and Diagnosis of the Infertile Male

5.4.1 History and Physical Examination

A lot of useful information can be obtained by taking a detailed history from the male partner and by performing a genital examination, although the latter may require some specific training. It is not unusual to pick up associated medical issues that may require further management and, increasingly, men are expecting that this be performed. In heterosexual couples, it is important to remember that there are two patients and female factors might determine what the ultimate management strategy might be.

Table 5.1 summarises some key questions for a simple medical history of the male that the gynaecologist or reproductive medicine specialist may find useful. The responses to each will alert the clinician to a possible problem that may require further evaluation. Importantly, however, it should be noted that many men may not remember (or even be aware) of some procedures (e.g. orchidopexy) that may have been performed in infancy. While partners can be an invaluable source of information, they can also be a hindrance to the taking of an accurate medical history, particularly if the male is too embarrassed to answer some questions honestly. The clinician should be mindful of this. Many men have reported the feeling of being 'side-lined' in a fertility consultation and therefore it is important to make them feel 'welcome' and 'involved'.

For all men a physical examination is recommended, although is often very rarely performed in a reproductive medicine setting (particularly if the results of semen analysis are normal) yet the initial perception of a patient can provide useful information. Some studies report a link between obesity and impaired semen quality. There is no doubt of a link between obesity, type 2 diabetes and impaired sexual function. Conversely, exaggerated muscular development could suggest that the patient may be using steroids. The average height of a person with

Table 5.1 A suggested questionnaire for undertaking a simple medical history of the male

Section 1: Fertility history

How long has he/they been trying to conceive (in months)?
Has he fathered any children before?

Section 2: Testicular/genital problems:

Does he have a history of any scrotal/groin procedures, injuries and/or infections (including sexually transmitted infections)?

Section 3: General medical and surgical history

Does he have a history of exposure to potentially gonadotoxic treatment, such as chemotherapy or radiotherapy?
Is there a history of surgery or trauma to the pelvis or abdomen, resulting in potential damage to the nerves that regulate sexual function?
Does he have a spinal cord injury?
Does he have a neurological disorder (including diabetes)?
Does he have any condition causing chronic ill health?
Is there an undiagnosed endocrinopathy?
Did he go through puberty at a normal age?
Does he shave infrequently?

Section 4: Drug history

Is he taking prescribed drugs, such those that can affect sexual functioning, such as antidepressants or antihypertensives?
Does he take over the counter drugs including herbal preparations?
Is he a user of illicit or recreational drugs, including cannabis?

Section 5: Family history

Is there a family history of anything that could affect fertility (e.g. cystic fibrosis, Kallman's syndrome)?

Section 6: Sexual history

Does he report any problems with libido, erections, orgasm or ejaculation?

Section 7: Lifestyle and environmental factors

Does he take steroids or protein supplements as part of bodybuilding or a fitness regime?
Does he undertake excessive exercise (e.g. triathlons)?
Does he wear tight-fitting underwear or skinny jeans?

Klinefelter syndrome is a little above average and this diagnosis can be considered in a young man with a tall slim build and low volume testes. Gynaecomastia is linked to endocrinopathies and can also be seen more commonly in men with Klinefelter syndrome.

Scrotal examination is a key part of the assessment but an understanding of what is 'normal' is of course key to this. The testes should on palpation feel smooth and firm. If hard or irregular lumps are detected an urgent ultrasound examination should be requested as testes cancer, although rare, is up to three times more common in subfertile men. The testes volume should be more than 15 mL and an orchidometer should be available in clinic to assess this. Low-volume or soft testes are associated with impaired sperm production and hypogonadism.

Occasionally the testes cannot be palpated, and, in these cases, an attempt should be made to locate them in the groin or inguinal areas. Groin ultrasonography or even magnetic resonance imaging of the abdomen and pelvis may be needed to locate the testes and confirm that it is structurally normal (undescended testes have an increased risk of malignancy). The vasa deferens are usually located at the postero-lateral aspect of the spermatic cord and feel like electric cables. Practice is required to get proficient in finding them, but bilateral absence is linked to carriage of CF gene mutations. Unilateral absence has a lower risk of being CF-related and may be due to a mesodermal developmental abnormality, which can also be responsible for an absent ipsilateral kidney. CF testing is mandatory in all men with vasal absence and then their partners, if a mutation is proven, to ensure that there is no significant risk of producing a child with mutations on both alleles and therefore clinical features of CF.

The epididymides can appear swollen or tender if affected by cysts or infection. Scrotal pain can also be caused by previous surgery. Varicoceles are best evaluated with the patient in the standing position and performing the Valsalva manoeuvre. Typically they diminish when the patient lies flat. If they do not, then (especially if the varicocele is on the less common right side), an abdominal ultrasound scan should be considered to exclude the rare possibility that the varicocele has been caused by a retroperitoneal lesion. Varicoceles can be assigned one of three grades: grade 1 (palpable only if patient performs a Valsalva manoeuvre), grade 2 (palpable, but not visible) and grade 3 (visible). It is generally believed that it is the larger (grades 2 and 3) clinical varicoceles that are relevant. Subclinical varicoceles that can be identified only on ultrasound scan are probably of no clinical significance.

5.4.2 Semen Analysis

Semen analysis is often seen as the first laboratory test that should be performed on the male, since it is relatively easy to perform, largely inexpensive and can quickly identify a number of important sperm-related issues that are a barrier to conception. However, if performed incorrectly, misdiagnosis can result very easily, so it is critical that clinicians refer their patients to a properly skilled and equipped laboratory with appropriate accreditation.

Guidelines for the laboratory examination of human semen have been published for many years by the World Health Organization [4] and these recommend the laboratory measurements that should be made. These are summarised in Table 5.2 along with the current reference ranges. It should be noted that the reference ranges are the fifth centile of a fertile population of men who achieved pregnancy with their partner within 12 months. They do not provide any information about the probability of success in assisted reproduction.

Men should be advised to abstain from ejaculation (by intercourse or masturbation) for between 2 and 7 days prior to the semen analysis being performed. This is so that the testicular output between men can be compared. Generally a single (normal) test result is adequate for clinical decision making, but it is controversial whether or not an abnormal test result should be repeated. If a repeat test is requested, then this should be performed at least 3 months after the first in order to allow for a full cycle of spermatogenesis to have been completed.

For men where retrograde ejaculation is suspected, special provision needs to be made for them to collect their post-masturbatory urine, after they have undergone a short period (several hours) of urinary alkalisation. Diagnostic laboratories should have protocols in place to deal with this and provide the male with written

Table 5.2 The World Health Organization recommended measurements of human semen and the associated reference values

Variable	Fifth centile (95% confidence Interval)
Semen volume (mL)	1.5 (1.4–1.7)
Sperm concentration ($\times 10^6$/mL)	15 (12–16)
Total sperm number ($\times 10^6$)	39 (33–46)
Progressive motility (%)	32 (31–34)
Total motility (%)	40 (38–42)
Vitality (% alive)	58 (55–63)
Normal morphology (%)	4 (3–4)

instructions about how to prepare for this test. Urine samples need to be examined quite quickly for the presence of sperm and therefore in such cases, urine and any semen samples provided normally need to be produced in a room close to the diagnostic laboratory.

5.4.3 Sperm Function Tests

One of the main criticisms of semen analysis is that it only describes in blunt terms the quantity and quality of sperm production, and in turn only broadly correlates with the probability of success either naturally or in assisted reproduction [5]. As such, there have been many tests developed to examine the functional aspects of sperm more closely (Table 5.3) including the assessment of sperm DNA integrity. However, to date, these have not been widely adopted and at the present time most professional bodies do not recommend their use [6].

5.4.4 Endocrine Tests

If semen analysis is abnormal, a baseline FSH (and testosterone) are helpful in placing the patient into a mechanistic category (Table 5.4). If the FSH and testosterone levels are low, then the rest of the pituitary hormones should be checked. If there are concerns about a pituitary tumour then a pituitary MRI should be discussed with an endocrinologist. Prolactin should be checked if there are symptoms related to hyperprolactinaemia, such as sexual dysfunction or breast symptoms of visual field defects.

5.4.5 Genetic Tests

Genetic testing in male infertility is currently of limited value and genetic factors are only identified in a small minority of men. However, it is important to perform, as some genetic issues have health implications for male patients and for any children whom they have. At the moment, the main genetic tests undertaken are karotyping, Y microdeletion testing and cystic fibrosis testing.

Karyotyping is used to look for chromosomal abnormalities such as duplications, deletions and translocations. Many guidelines advocate testing karyotype in men with a sperm concentration of less than 10 million/mL, but the chance of finding an abnormality increases with the severity of the reduction in sperm concentration, so only about 10%–15% of men with non-obstructive azo-ospermia (NOA) are

Table 5.3 A summary of sperm function tests

	Commonly used	Some current use	Largely obsolete
Microscopy			
Semen analysis	✓		
Hypo-osmotic swelling test		✓	
Sperm morphology measurements	✓		
Sperm movement			
Computer-assisted sperm analysis		✓	
Sperm hyperactivation			✓
Sperm–cervical mucus interaction			
Sperm–cervical mucus contact test			✓
Kramer test			✓
Post-coital test			✓
Sperm capacitation assessment			
Acrosin activity			✓
Acrosome integrity			✓
Acrosome reaction			✓
Cap Score (percentage of fertilization-competent, capacitated spermatozoa)		✓	
Sperm egg binding assessment			
Sperm–zona interaction			✓
Sperm–oolemma binding			✓
Zona free hamster oocyte test			✓
Hyaluronan binding assay		✓	
Oxidative stress			
Reactive oxygen species levels		✓	
Total antioxidant capacity		✓	
Sperm DNA quality			
Sperm DNA fragmentation		✓	
Chromatin compaction		✓	

found to have an abnormal karyotype. The most common abnormal finding in men with NOA is Klinefelter syndrome (XXY). Other findings may increase the risk of miscarriage or fetal abnormality and when an abnormal karyotype is found, genetic counselling should be considered.

Y microdeletion testing should be performed on men who have a sperm concentration of less than 5 million/mL as well as in cases of idiopathic azoospermia, or prior to surgical sperm retrieval. Where AZFa, AZFb or a mixed genotype containing one of these mutations is found, surgical sperm retrieval should not be performed and men should be advised to consider other forms of family formation such as donor insemination, adoption or fostering. In a small number of men with AZFc, low concentrations of sperm may be seen in the ejaculate and in up to 60% of the remainder, sperm can be recovered surgically. It is important to advise the couple that if sperm are recovered and a son is born, it is almost certain he will inherit the same Y chromosome microdeletion and therefore have fertility problems when he becomes an adult. Daughters are unaffected. Y microdeletions are an indication for pre-implantation genetic diagnosis (PGD) in some countries, but not in the United Kingdom.

CF testing is mandatory in (1) cases of azoospermia with vasal absence on examination, (2) men with a family history of cystic fibrosis or (3) where, on assessment, patients have clinical features of CF. It should also be tested if the partner is known to have either CF or to be a carrier. If both partners are carriers then PGD can be considered.

Table 5.4 Endocrine measurements in men

	FSH	Testosterone
Pre-testicular		
Hypothalamic/ pituitary failure	Low	low
Anabolic steroid usage	Very low	Normal or high[a]
Testicular		
Isolated spermatogenesis defect	High (usually)[b]	Normal
Primary hypogonadism	High	Low
Post-testicular		
Obstructive azoospermia	Normal	Normal

[a] The same result can be seen in testosterone-secreting tumours, which are extraordinarily rare.
[b] In late maturation arrest, which can occur in up to 20% of cases of non-obstructive azo-ospermia, as the trigger for inhibin B release occurs prior to the arrest point in spermatogenetic arrest, the brain falsely interprets the normal Inhibin B levels as meaning that sperm is being made. This is why a normal FSH level does not always mean male genital tract obstruction.

5.4.6 Radiological Investigations

Scrotal ultrasonography should be arranged on an urgent basis if, at physical examination, there is a concern about testicular tumour or considered if a clinical varicocele is detected. Groin/abdominal ultrasound scans can also be performed to locate undescended testes, prior to urological referral. Undescended testes have a 2- to 5-fold increased risk of becoming cancerous and a scan at this point can (if the testes are visible), exclude this possibility. Abdominal and pelvic MRI scans are required in men whose testes cannot be located on ultrasound scan. Transrectal ultrasound scanning (or MRI) can be used to investigate men to exclude ejaculatory duct obstruction. Such men are azoospermic, with a normal hormone profile and a low volume ejaculate. They may report pain on ejaculation. Vasography can be considered to exclude a proximal blockage if vasal reconstructive surgery is being performed.

5.4.7 Other Investigations

On occasions it is helpful to screen men for genital infections and not just when their partner has a positive test. If the semen analysis result shows persistent numbers of white blood cells, semen and urine samples should be sent for culture and STI screening performed or recommended. Testing for sperm antibodies is generally not recommended [5]; neither is performing testicular biopsies for purposes of histological characterisation only. The latter is not strongly predictive of outcome and unless testicular neoplasia needs to be excluded, histological biopsies should be performed only as part of a surgical sperm retrieval procedure.

5.5 Treatment Options

5.5.1 Medical Management

In cases of secondary hypogonadism, GnRH replacement is challenging due to the technical nature of pumps that can replicate the natural pulsatile release, and so pituitary hormone replacement is the norm. Various protocols exist that essentially involve replacing LH with human chorionic gonadotropin (hCG) and assessing the response to treatment by monitoring testicular volume and testosterone levels [7]. Generally, patients get to their maximum testosterone level within 2 years. When testosterone levels normalise, and there is no further increase in testes volume, human menopausal gonadotropin or recombinant FSH can then be added to replace FSH and semen analysis subsequently performed to assess fertility. hCG monotherapy can be effective in milder cases. The more severe cases (testes volume <4 mL) have a lower chance of achieving spermatogenesis. The side effects can include gynaecomastia due to increased oestrogen levels. Some experts advocate FSH pre-treatment in men who have not gone through puberty. If the couple become pregnant then the treatment can be discontinued in the second trimester (in case of miscarriage) and the man switched to testosterone. If the sperm quality does not reach a quality at which natural conception is likely, then samples can be stored and used for ICSI. Sperm storage should also be considered if pituitary hormone replacement therapy is going to end.

With the exception of hormone replacement therapy for conditions that are caused by a deficiency of hypothalamic or pituitary hormones, there is limited evidence that drugs such as clomifene, hCG, aromatase inhibitors and tamoxifen can improve sperm production. Clomifene can be used as a fertility-sparing alternative to testosterone replacement therapy, to boost endogenous testosterone production in men who are symptomatic of hypogonadism.

In recent years, there has been increasing interest in whether over-the-counter or prescribed formulations of nutritional supplements for men can boost sperm production. Their use is largely based on small randomised trials on various formulations, doses and durations. The most recent meta-analysis [8] to examine these data suggests that there is very little evidence of benefit in terms of increasing the chances of pregnancy, even though small marginal gains in sperm quality can be shown (compared to placebo). As such, there is insufficient evidence currently to recommend the use of these supplements.

5.5.2 Surgical Management

Surgical management can be considered in cases of (1) clinical varicocele, (2) prior vasectomy and (3) ejaculatory duct obstruction, as described in the text that follows.

For men with a clinical varicocele, most studies have shown that varicocele treatment improves semen parameters and also sperm DNA fragmentation rates and others, including randomised controlled trials, have shown an improvement in natural pregnancy rates. However, the results from meta-analyses have not been conclusive, owing in part to the nature of the studies that were included and the variability of their design and selection criteria [9]. The impact of varicocele treatment on surgical sperm retrieval for NOA is less certain and further studies are needed to clarify this. However, treatment can be considered on a case by case basis in couples with proven infertility and a clinical varicocele associated with impaired semen quality, or in men with testicular pain that is believed to be linked to the varicocele (although varicoceles are generally painless). Varicocele treatment can be performed by angiographic embolization or surgical ligation. Sub-inguinal microsurgical varicocele ligation is associated with the highest cure rates and has the lowest complication rates of the surgical approaches.

In cases of men who have previously had a vasectomy, a vasovasostomy can be considered. The best results are obtained if the procedure is done within 7 years of the original vasectomy, using a microsurgical approach, and in situations in which the female partner is younger and has no female fertility problems. The chance of success diminishes particularly after 15 years, due to chronic fibrosis. It is contraindicated in cases of tubal infertility in the female partner and in such circumstances; men should be offered surgical sperm retrieval with ICSI. As an alternative, vaso-epididymostomy (anastomosing the vas to the epididymal tubule) can be performed in cases of epididymal obstruction, but this has significantly worse outcomes.

In the rare circumstance of ejaculatory duct obstruction, the obstructed ducts can be resected endoscopically (transurethral resection of ejaculatory ducts) to facilitate natural conception and avoid surgical sperm retrieval and ICSI. The potential adverse effects of this procedure can include urinary incontinence and restenosis. The patients frequently report 'watery' ejaculate.

5.5.3 Assisted Reproduction

For many years, the only form of assisted reproduction for men with poor fertility (of any cause) was to consider the use of donor sperm. Whilst this is still an option for azoospermic men where sperm is not recovered at surgical sperm recovery (or where they choose to use it for other reasons), donor sperm is now used less often by heterosexual couples due to the advent of ICSI (see later).

Today perhaps the simplest form of assisted reproduction for male subfertility is intra-uterine insemination (IUI). This is where ejaculated (or frozen/thawed) sperm obtained is washed (see Chapter 9 for details) and then inseminated into the female partner immediately prior to ovulation. This can achieve reasonable success rates (after a half dozen attempts a typically quoted cumulative live birth rate would be in excess of 50%) and for some men (e.g. those with spinal injuries or retrograde ejaculation) can provide a cost-effective treatment. However, its use has come under greater scrutiny in recent years and in cases of unexplained infertility (i.e. where sperm quality is normal) it probably is no more successful than expectant management [10].

While in vitro fertilisation was initially developed to help in cases of infertility caused by tubal blockage in the female partner, it was quickly modified in a number of ways to try and enhance the fertilising ability of sperm that were poorly motile or simply too few in number. This led to the development of ICSI, where individual sperm are injected into the cytoplasm of eggs recovered from the female partner (or donor). Details of the laboratory procedures involved in ICSI are outlined elsewhere in this book (see Chapter 9), so the primary focus here is to briefly outline the various procedures that can be used to recover sperm, depending on the nature of the underlying problem.

In cases of obstructive azoospermia, sperm may be recovered by either an 'aspiration procedure' or an 'open testicular procedure' largely depending on the clinician's preference and training. There is a very high chance of getting sperm in cases of obstructive azo-ospermia (almost 100%), but the amount of sperm recovered differs between the procedures.

Aspiration procedures include (1) percutaneous epididymal sperm aspiration (PESA), in which a fine needle is passed into the epididymis percutaneously and the aspirated fluid examined for sperm; (2) microsurgical epididymal sperm aspiration (MESA), which is performed via an open incision to allow direct visualisation of the epididymis under an operating microscope; or (3) testicular sperm aspiration (TESA), in which a small biopsy of testicular issue is recovered from the testicle through a small needle attached to a syringe. In each case, these are generally performed under local anaesthetic and are carried out as an outpatient procedure, although MESA is generally performed under general anaesthesia.

Open testicular procedures are termed testicular sperm extraction (TESE) and are either single site (usually performed under local anaesthetic) or multisite (usually requiring a general anaesthetic).

In cases of non-obstructive azoospermia microTESE is considered the gold standard procedure. In this procedure, the testes are opened and the parenchyma examined under an operating microscope, to look for differences in tubule diameter that predict complete spermatogenesis. The procedure can be lengthy, but typical recovery rates are in the region of 50%.

The sperm recovered from surgical sperm recovery can be used either immediately (i.e. fresh) or can be frozen for future use. However, studies show variable success in using frozen sperm and so careful consideration should be given to the timing of the procedure depending on the preference of the IVF laboratory for the use of fresh or frozen sperm.

5.6 Concluding Remarks

In conclusion, the appropriate assessment and management of the infertile male is an important and often overlooked aspect of reproductive medicine. However, as outlined in this chapter, there are several aspects of care which can be simply delivered by the gynaecologist or reproductive medicine specialist in a general setting.

References

1. El Osta R, Almont T, Diligent C, Hubert N, Eschwège P, Hubert J. Anabolic steroids abuse and male infertility. *Basic Clin Androl*. 2016;**26**:2. DOI: 10.1186/s12610-016-0029-4.

2. Eley A, Pacey AA, Galdiero M, Galdiero M, Galdiero F. Can *Chlamydia trachomatis* directly damage your sperm? *Lancet Infect Dis*. 2005;**5**:53–7.

3. Povey AC, Clyma JA, McNamee R, Moore HD, Baillie H, Pacey AA, Cherry NM; Participating Centres of Chaps-UK. Modifiable and non-modifiable risk factors for poor semen quality: a case referent study. *Hum Reprod*. 2012;**27**:2799–806.

4. World Health Organization. *WHO laboratory manual for the examination and processing of human semen*, 5th ed. Geneva: World Health Organization; 2010.

5. Tomlinson M, Lewis S, Morroll D; British Fertility Society. Sperm quality and its relationship to natural and assisted conception: British Fertility Society guidelines for practice. *Hum Fertil (Camb)*. 2013;**16**:175–93. DOI: 10.3109/14647273.2013.807522.

6. Pacey A. Is sperm DNA fragmentation a useful test that identifies a treatable cause of male infertility? *Best Pract Res Clin Obstet Gynaecol*. 2018;**53**:11–19.

7. Prior M, Stewart J, McEleny K, Dwyer AA, Quinton R. Fertility induction in hypogonadotropic hypogonadal men. *Clin Endocrinol (Oxf)*. 2018;**89**:712–18.

8. Smits RM, Mackenzie-Proctor R, Yazdani A, Stankiewicz MT, Jordan V, Showell MG. Antioxidants for male subfertility. *Cochrane Database Syst Rev*. 2019; (**3**): CD007411. DOI: 10.1002/14651858.CD007411.pub4.

9. Yan S, Shabbir M, Yap T, Homa S, Ramsay J, McEleny K, Minhas S. Should the current guidelines for the treatment of varicoceles in infertile men be re-evaluated? *Hum Fertil (Camb)*. 2019; (in press).

10. Veltman-Verhulst SM, Hughes E, Ayeleke RO, Cohlen BJ. Intra-uterine insemination for unexplained subfertility. *Cochrane Database Syst Rev*. 2016;Feb **19**; (2):CD001838. DOI: 10.1002/14651858.CD001838.pub5.

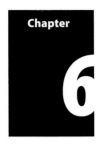

Chapter

6

Unexplained Infertility

Ben Willem Mol and Andrew William Nguyen

6.1 Introduction

Infertility, which refers to failure to conceive within one year of having regular unprotected intercourse, occurs in one of every six couples [1]. Infertility can broadly be categorised into tubal pathology, anovulation, reduced sperm quality and unexplained infertility.

From planning pregnancy to eventually seeking treatment for infertility, couples tend to follow a typical pattern of progression. In those desiring pregnancy, approximately 84% will have natural conception within the first 12 months of unprotected intercourse [2]. A proportion of unsuccessful couples then go on to seek fertility assistance. Generally, the typical fertility consultation involves conducting a comprehensive history and examination of the couple to determine if there is a medical cause for which the infertility can be attributed. Fertility investigations follow focusing on whether the gametes can meet each other, namely to identify issues with semen, ovulation and transport, that is, tubal patency or the pelvic cavity [3]. Following the work-up, only about 60% of cases have an identifiable cause and lead to a diagnosis of male and/or female subfertility, while the other 40% have no detected abnormalities, leading them to be labelled as so-called unexplained infertility [4].

There is consensus among the European Society of Reproductive Medicine (ESHRE) and National Institute for Health and Care Excellence (NICE) in their guidelines for infertility treatment that couples first be informed about their chances of spontaneous conception and consequently not be subjected to treatments that are ineffective or pose needless potential harm [3, 5]. Before a treatment is initiated, it must be determined whether it is appropriate for the specific couple and if potential benefits offset the risks of harm. Couples with regular cycles post-fertility work-up can have their probability for natural conception estimated using the Hunault synthesis prediction

model [6, 7]. For couples with unexplained subfertility with low likelihood for spontaneous conception, medically assisted reproduction becomes warranted when treatment is expected to improve chances of achieving pregnancy above their chance naturally [3]. The rationale for which treatment should be approached is to view it in terms of prognosis rather than diagnosis; the question becomes 'what will occur in the near future?' as opposed to 'what is causing the infertility?'.

6.2 Prediction Models

6.2.1 History of Prediction Models

To date, there are nine published prediction models pertaining to natural conception in infertile couples [6, 8, 9–13]. The first model was developed in 1993 by Bostofte et al. in a Danish cohort utilising three variables: subfertility duration; sperm penetration test and type of female subfertility, which could either be none, ovulatory or cervical condition, an anatomical issue or a mixture of conditions [8]. Most recently, a group in the Netherlands developed the synthesis model using combined data from the cohorts of the Snick, Collins and Eimers studies [9–11]. The synthesis model of Hunault et al. considers a number of different variables, namely female age, subfertility duration, whether subfertility is primary or secondary, percentage sperm motility, whether referral was by a specialist gynaecologist or general practitioner and optionally the post-coital test results [6].

At present, no current fertility treatment guidelines promote the use of prediction models to guide clinical practice, with perhaps one contributing factor being that validation within external populations of such prediction models has only recently occurred [14]. Table 6.1 summarises the different prognostic factors used in different research models to predict natural conception in couples with infertility.

Table 6.1 A comparison of natural conception prediction models for infertile couples

Authors	Prognostic factors

Bostofte et al. (1993) [8]	• Duration of infertility
	• Infertility factor (classified in this study as):
	  o Normal
	  o Ovulation
	  o Anatomical or cervical
	  o Combination
	• Sperm penetration test (P-test)

Eimers et al. (1994) [11]	• Duration of infertility • Primary or secondary infertility • Percentage (%) sperm motility in first semen analysis • Post-coital test (first) results
Bahamondes et al. (1994) [12]	• Sperm morphology • Age of female partner • Duration of infertility • Primary or secondary infertility • Female partner history of pelvic surgery • Menstrual cycle duration
Wichmann et al. (1994) [13]	• Duration of infertility • Age of both male and female partner • History of male urethritis • Body mass index • % sperm motility • Motility quality • Motile sperm density • Total motile count • Sperm morphology • Semen pH
Collins et al. (1995) [10]	• Pregnancy history • Duration of infertility • Age of female partner • Presence of male defect • Endometriosis • Tubal disease
Snick et al. (1997) [9]	• Duration of infertility • Post-coital test results • Tubal disease • Ovulation issue
Hunault et al. (2004) – Synthesis model [6]	• Duration of infertility • Age of female partner • Primary or secondary infertility • Total motile sperm concentration • Referral status, i.e. referred by general practitioner or gynaecologist

6.2.2 Performance of the Synthesis Model for Natural Conception

The limitation in many predictive models is that conclusions drawn are largely specific to the population in which the model was developed, with overly optimistic outcomes being drawn when employed in populations which differ from the original [15]. As such, both internal and external validation of any prediction model should be conducted before considering use in clinical practice [16, 17].

Internal validation involves utilising the population on which the prediction model is based to determine what would constitute over-optimistic estimates and consequently adjust the model accordingly. Unlike with previous models, the more recent predictive models have had internal validation applied [8, 11–13]. When assessing prediction models, however, external validation is of greater practical value given that the model can be prospectively applied in a different population than that in which it was developed, albeit at great financial cost and with significant time consumption [16].

The process of external validation was applied to the Hunault natural conception prediction model, which demonstrated that the model's calibration was nearly flawless [7]. The study population involved 3,000 subfertile couples, 537 (18%) of whom had spontaneous ongoing pregnancy, 55 (2%) had pregnancy loss, 1,316 (44%) commenced treatment, 820 (27%) were neither pregnant nor initiated treatment and 280 (9%) were lost to follow-up. Cumulative ongoing pregnancy rates in couples with prognosis ≥40% was 46% without treatment, which paralleled the discriminative capacity of the original sample population in which the model was based (c-statistic: 0.59).

Despite there being a common tendency to dwell on the principle of discrimination (differentiating between those who will and will not spontaneously conceive), the emphasis should be on determining the likelihood that a couple will conceive. Approached from this context, improvements can be made on the current Hunault prediction model by incorporating further prognostic factors such as a couple's comprehensive fertility history, the woman's body mass index (BMI), cycle duration, basal follicle-stimulating hormone (FSH) level and a semen analysis. Additional potential prognostic factors were explored in the analysis of an extended cohort [7, 18]. Factors which enhanced prediction of natural conception include history of pregnancy within current relationship, cycle duration, BMI, sperm volume, concentration and World Health Organization (WHO) morphology. Figure 6.1 depicts the additional prognostic indicators used in conjunction with those in the Hunault synthesis model for natural conception for infertile couples.

6.3 Treatment of Unexplained Infertility

At present, the likelihood of conceiving can be naturally predicted for couples with unexplained infertility, which leads to the clinical question of which couples should be treated and when this should occur. The two predominant methods employed in the treatment of unexplained infertility are intrauterine insemination (IUI) with or without ovarian stimulation and in vitro fertilisation (IVF).

6.3.1 Intrauterine Insemination

The process of IUI begins with monitoring of the ovulatory cycle with ultrasound or urine testing for the luteinizing hormone (LH) surge. When ovulation is anticipated, the insemination is planned. This starts with processing of semen through laboratory 'washing', such that motile spermatozoa can be prepared and concentrated into a small volume for delivery into the uterus. Sperm is delivered directly into the uterine cavity via a small catheter, thereby bypassing the cervix entirely. The premise of IUI is to increase the likelihood of fertilisation by delivering the sperm into the uterus such that it is in close proximity to the released oocyte. The success of IUI is critically dependent on coinciding the procedure with ovulation; hence cycle monitoring is employed to determine timing precisely.

Additional means of improving timing of IUI with ovulation is to perform it together with mild ovarian hyperstimulation (MOH). MOH is typically achieved through use of clomiphene citrate (CC), letrozole or subcutaneous injection of gonadotropins. The premise of MOH is to improve accuracy of timing and to increase the number of oocytes available to be fertilised. Comparisons between IUI (with or without MOH) efficacy relative to expectant management have been drawn and it is a topic currently fiercely debated with no unanimous consensus. Concerns have been expressed regarding multiple pregnancy rates when IUI is augmented with MOH. A recent Cochrane review comprising 14 trials with a total population size of 1,867 women failed to demonstrate that women with unexplained infertility treated with IUI (irrespective of MOH use) compared to expectant management or timed intercourse differed significantly in terms of rates of live birth or multiple pregnancy [19]. The treatment effect is likely to be dependent on prognosis. While in couples with a poor prognosis for natural conception MOH IUI seems to have additional value, its additional effect in women with good prospects for natural conception is limited [20, 21].

6.3.2 In Vitro Fertilisation

IVF use has expanded over the years and it has been increasingly utilised in all causes of subfertility despite there being a distinct lack of data regarding efficacy in such cases. Together with the mounting evidence of IVF use being associated with adverse health

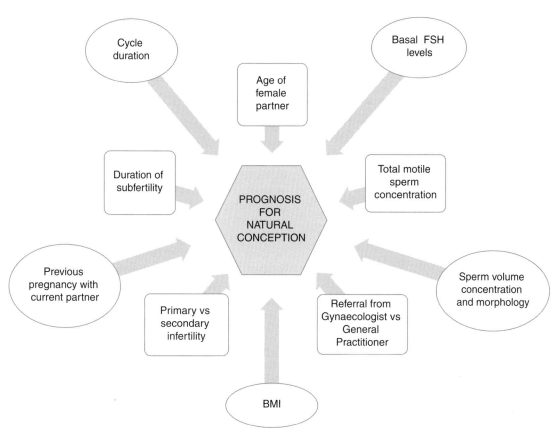

Figure 6.1 Prognostic factors for predicting natural conception in couples with subfertility. The likelihood of conceiving within one year can be predicted using various prognostic factors. Factors chosen in the Hunault synthesis model (boxes) have been externally validated and have shown good predictive capability for estimating the chance for natural spontaneous conception. Additional prognostic factors (circled), when combined with the Hunault synthesis model, have shown greater predictive capability than the synthesis model alone. BMI, body mass index; FSH, follicle-stimulating hormone.

outcomes in children born through such means, a frank discussion must be had regarding its use.

Conducting IVF involves a standard regimen, notably beginning with controlled ovarian stimulation (COS), followed by oocyte retrieval under ultrasound guidance, laboratory insemination, culturing of embryo/s and lastly transcervical replacement of embryos during either the cleavage or blastocyst stage. IVF is an invasive therapy that does carry risk for numerous complications, including multiple pregnancy and ovarian hyperstimulation syndrome (OHSS). Despite its risks, use of IVF in unexplained infertility may be warranted to overcome unknown biological shortcomings contributing to infertility by bypassing various in vivo steps which may be impairing the ability to conceive. Such factors may include ovarian dysfunction, cervical factors, issues with sperm and egg transport and sperm–egg interaction.

Hughes et al. conducted a randomised controlled trial (RCT) comparing IVF with expectant management [22]. The trial involved 139 couples and compared one cycle of IVF with 3 months expectant management, with results demonstrating higher live birth rates in the IVF-treated group. The evidence presented in the study, however, was considered to be low quality [23]. In particular, the average duration of subfertility among the patients was 4 years, which is a long duration relative to other studies drawing comparisons between treatment and expectant management in unexplained infertility. Furthermore, prospective studies have demonstrated that timed intercourse must be undertaken across a minimum of six cycles, not simply 3 months, to adequately cover the interval in which the majority of conceptions theoretically occur [24].

6.3.3 Treatments Preceding IUI and IVF

6.3.3.1 Tubal Flushing

Hysterosalpingography (HSG) refers to a diagnostic technique used to assess tubal patency that has been commonly used in the outpatient setting for this purpose since the establishment of the method in 1914. There has been speculation since the 1950s that potential fertility benefits are linked to HSGs, whereby the act of flushing tubes directly contributes to increased rates of pregnancy in the months post-procedure. Numerous studies have since demonstrated fertility benefits are derived specifically from HSG using oil-based contrast mediums; however, only three such studies were RCTs [26–28]. Analysis of pooled data from the RCTs suggested higher ongoing pregnancy rates in women who received an HSG with oil-based contrast relative to no intervention (odds ratio [OR] 3.6; 95% confidence interval [CI] 2.1–6.3) [29]. A meta-analysis was conducted to compare how different types of HSG contrasts, notably oil- and water-based contrast, differ in terms of pregnancy rates [29]. The analysis included five RCTs and demonstrated that although there were higher ongoing pregnancy rates in the oil-based group compared to the water-based groups, the results were not statistically significant (OR 1.4; 95% CI 0.8–2.5). There should be caution with regards to interpretation of these results, given the studies included in the meta-analysis were deemed low-quality studies associated with a large degree of uncertainty regarding the result estimates.

Given the ambiguity surrounding the effects of the two different HSG contrasts on pregnancy rates, a multicentre trial [30] randomised infertile women were randomised to HSG tubal flushing with either oil-based contrast medium (Lipiodol®) or water-based contrast medium (Telebrix Hystero®). The trial demonstrated both higher ongoing pregnancy rates (39.7% vs. 29.1%, respectively) and live birth rates (38.8% vs. 28.1%) in those receiving oil-based contrast.

6.3.3.2 Lifestyle Interventions

Obesity undoubtedly constitutes a large public health issue overall, especially if one considers that 20% of reproductive-aged women in developed nations are obese, but it also specifically impacts women desiring pregnancy given associations between obesity and anovulation, menstrual abnormalities and infertility in general [31–35]. Numerous guidelines on infertility treatment of obese women recommend the first step of management is to aim for a 5%–10% reduction of their weight [36, 37]. Despite such a recommendation being quite commonplace, there is a noticeable scarcity in studies investigating the impact on pregnancy outcomes with effective weight loss in accordance with recommended goals.

A multicentre RCT of comprising 577 obese infertile women aged between 18 and 39 [38] involved randomisation of 290 women to a 6-month lifestyle programme followed by 18 months of fertility treatment and the remaining 287 women to immediate fertility treatment over 24 months. Fertility treatment used in the study occurred as per Dutch infertility guidelines, with women being assigned treatment modalities based on presence of anovulation, the natural conception prognosis as per the Hunault synthesis model and by what treatments they had failed in the past. Women in this study thereby received treatment with ovulation induction, expectant management, IUI, and/or IVF or intracytoplasmic sperm injection (ICSI). With number of vaginal deliveries of healthy, term singletons at 24 months following randomisation used as the outcome, it was found that the intervention group had a significantly smaller proportion of births than the control groups (27.1% vs. 35.2%), with the rate ratio being 0.77 (95% CI 0.60–0.99). However, there was a significantly larger proportion of women with an ongoing pregnancy who conceived naturally in the intervention group (26.1%) than in the control group (16.2%), with the rate ratio being 1.61 (95% CI 1.16–2.24).

6.4 The Preferred Path: Comparative Assessment of First-Line Treatments

Four treatment domains come into play when considering the first-line therapy of choice to use in couples with unexplained subfertility: effectiveness, safety, burden and costs.

6.4.1 Effectiveness

When contrasting the effectiveness of both first-line treatments in unexplained infertility, the outcome is naturally measured by the ability for couples to have a live birth. Delivery rates with IUI (with MOH) is approximately 8% per cycle, compared to the 29% pregnancy rate which has been demonstrated with IVF [39]. While RCTs conducted on females aged between 18 and 38 with unexplained infertility have demonstrated higher per cycle pregnancy rates in IVF relative to IUI, no significant differences are observed in cumulative pregnancy rates over 12 months in treatment-naïve couples undergoing a maximum of six cycles of either IUI (with or without MOH) or IVF, or in one cycle of IVF with elective single embryo transfer compared to three cycles of IUI [40, 41].

6.4.2 Safety

Safety as it relates to treatment primarily has to do with potential for physical harm, which can manifest in the context of unexplained infertility as maternal or neonatal complications. The primary concern in IUI or IVF is the increased risk of multiple pregnancy, which has been estimated to be 7% with IUI and 19% in IVF [39]. Those multiple pregnancies which lead to two or more at or near full-term healthy babies do not technically present an issue. However, the potential for increased adverse maternal and neonatal complications and outcomes has prompted initiatives to reduce multiple pregnancy rates. Single embryo transfers (SETs) represent one such measure used to combat multiple pregnancy rates and have been adopted by a number of countries such as Australia, New Zealand, Scandinavia, Belgium and the Netherlands. Results from two RCTs demonstrated comparable multiple pregnancy rates in treatment-naïve couples receiving IUI and IVF with SET [40, 41]. IVF compares unfavourably to IUI, however, in terms of the former's risk of OHSS, which is rarely an issue for IUI even with MOS.

6.4.3 Burden

The concept of burden pertains to how receiving a treatment will affect a couple's overall wellbeing and functional capacity. The fertility treatments utilised in unexplained infertility have an accompanying physical burden, which is compounded given there is often a need for repeated visits to the fertility clinic. IUI and ovarian stimulation imposes a physical burden, as does IVF, which is generally more painful than the former given adverse effects from medication used in the stimulation phase, need for follicle aspiration and ovarian enlargement within the luteal phase. Burden is also present as psychological distress, commonly anxiety and depression, which is typically prominent during or after failed or cancelled treatments [42].

6.4.4 Costs

Costs represent an important consideration in treatment and are defined as the financial expenditure required to successfully achieve the outcome of interest. The cost of IVF is far greater than that of IUI in a comparison per cycle [43].

6.4.5 The Preferred Path?

Bearing in mind each of the four criteria which dictate first-line treatment, IUI with mild ovarian stimulation (MOH) is seemingly better given it carries less burden, has a greater safety profile, is less costly and appears to have approximately equal efficacy compared to IVF. Figure 6.2 summarises the characteristics of IUI and IVF across the four domains as they pertain to first-line treatment of unexplained infertility.

A recent trial sought to investigate if different methods of IVF – IVF with SET or IVF in a modified natural cycle – could have comparable live birth rates to IUI–COS while reducing multiple pregnancy rates in couples with unexplained infertility and poor prognosis for natural conception [44]. The findings demonstrated that, across all three groups, the number of couples who delivered healthy children after one year were comparable and that all groups had low multiple pregnancy rates. The main distinction between all these modalities is that both forms of IVF are substantially more expensive than IUI [45]. The INeS trial results have been widely used to support the effectiveness of IUI and justify it as appropriate first-line therapy [46]. Drawing such a conclusion may be unwarranted at this stage, however, given there are implicit suggestions that, first, IUI has proven superiority over no treatment, and second that IVF similarly has an advantage over sexual intercourse in couples with unexplained subfertility.

Figure 6.2 Comparison of first-line treatments in unexplained infertility. First-line treatments for unexplained infertility include intrauterine insemination (IUI) with or without controlled ovarian stimulation (COS) and in vitro fertilisation (IVF). When comparing IUI ± COS with IVF, effectiveness as measured by cumulative live birth rates is comparable among treatment-naïve couples across six cycles for each therapy, with the former also being safer, associated with less burden and having lower costs.

6.5 IUI and IVF Use in Unexplained Infertility: What's the Evidence?

6.5.1 IUI

6.5.1.1 IUI versus Sexual Intercourse

A recent review by the Cochrane Collaboration examined live birth rates in couples with unexplained infertility undergoing IUI, with or without controlled ovarian hyperstimulation (COS), compared to unprotected sexual intercourse in the presence or absence of cycle monitoring [19]. Three RCTs were identified by authors, which in total included a population of 690 couples with unexplained infertility of average duration 2–4 years, with females being on average 33 years old [47–49]. Among the three studies, only one compared IUI and timed sexual intercourse using cycle monitoring [47], while the other two studies contrasted IUI with sexual intercourse in the absence of medical co-interventions [48, 49]. Using the outcome of clinical pregnancy, a comparison between IUI without MOH relative to sexual intercourse demonstrated an OR of 1.53 (95% CI: 0.88–2.64), while IUI with COS in comparison to sexual intercourse was 1.00 (95% CI: 0.59–1.67). The OR for multiple pregnancy in IUI without COS compared to sexual intercourse was 0.50 (95% CI: 0.04–5.53), while for IUI with COS relative to sexual intercourse was 2.00 (95% CI: 0.18–22.34).

The conclusions inferred by the authors based on these results was that there is inconclusive evidence to support that there are differences in pregnancy outcomes between IUI, with or without COS, compared to sexual intercourse. Notably, the authors outlined the need to determine if multiple pregnancy rates after IUI could be lessened to an appropriate degree without compromising live birth rates, which could be achieved through contrasting IUI without COS to IUI with COS with low-dose gonadotropins.

6.5.1.2 The Trial on Intrauterine Insemination (TUI Study): Is IUI Better in Good or Bad Prognosis Couples?

A recent trial sought to investigate how outcomes differ between IUI and expectant management in a two-centre, open-label, RCT [20]. A total of 201 couples with unfavourable prognosis for natural conception were randomised for three cycles to either IUI with ovarian stimulation (using oral CC or oral letrozole) or expectant management. Of the 101 women who received IUI, there were 31 live births (31%),

compared to 9 (9%) live births in the 100 women receiving expectant management. The risk ratio for the outcome of live birth in IUI compared to expectant management was 3.41 (95% CI: 1.71–6.79), implying that the couples receiving IUI when they have poor prognosis in unexplained infertility have higher cumulative live birth rates and that the treatment is effective in this clinical context. Findings from a similar study, which differed from the above trial primarily in that couples had a favourable prognosis for natural conception (less than 2 years attempting to conceive), demonstrated that use of immediate IUI did not improve upon cumulative live birth rates from 6 months of expectant management [48].

6.5.2 IVF

6.5.2.1 IVF versus Sexual Intercourse

The Cochrane Collaboration similarly published a review comparing the efficacy and safety of IVF in treatment of unexplained infertility to sexual intercourse [17]. Only two relevant studies, both of which were RCTs, were identified by authors for this analysis [22]. In both original studies, only a subset of the population could be used in the Cochrane review, as not all the couples had a diagnosis of unexplained infertility. As such, the first study contributed 35 out of 245 couples while the second study had 51 of 139 couples who could be included in this analysis. The Cochrane review thereby had a total study size of 86 couples, in whom the average duration for trying to conceive was 5 years and the average female age was 33 years. In the first study, a comparison was drawn between one IVF cycle and 6 months of sexual intercourse with or without reproductive treatment excluding IVF. The second study similarly compared one IVF cycle, albeit to 90 days of sexual intercourse alone. Other outcome measures, such as rate of multiple pregnancy, OHSS, miscarriage or costs, were not reported on in these studies.

The two RCTs had results demonstrating opposing treatment effect directions, which suggests that a high degree of heterogeneity was present. For the outcome of clinical pregnancy in IVF compared to sexual intercourse, the first study had an OR of 0.30 (95% CI: 0.02–3.67), while the second study had an OR of 8.00 (95% CI: 1.89–33.85), leading to a pooled OR 3.24 (95% CI: 1.07–9.80). Considering the second study, given its apparent positive treatment effect, a considerable difference in conception rates (29% vs. 1%) seemingly implies IVF is an effective tool in subfertility treatment. Notably, the study population had average duration of subfertility exceeding 4 years, which is far longer than seen in many couples who seek IVF. Additionally, it is likely that there was a proportion of couples within this study who were included despite having conditions such as severe oligospermia, anovulation or severe endometriosis (American Fertility Society [AFS] class III or IV), which would make them ineligible for expectant management given the absent chance for conceiving spontaneously.

The authors' conclusion based on the pooled results of both studies is that there is inadequate evidence to suggest that IVF significantly provides better clinical pregnancy outcomes than sexual intercourse in unexplained infertility. The authors underscored that future directions should involve subsequent subfertility trials having concordant study designs, methods and result presentation such that data can be better pooled, in addition to having studies that investigate the timing at which the transition from sexual intercourse to invasive first-line treatment options should occur. Table 6.2 summarises the current literature comparing the efficacy of sexual intercourse to IUI and IVF in couples with unexplained infertility.

6.5.2.2 Is IVF Use Justifiable in Unexplained Subfertility?

IVF for use in tubal-factor infertility represents a situation whereby randomised trials to demonstrate treatment effectiveness are unwarranted, given the likelihood of spontaneous conception is low and the therapy can essentially circumvent the issue of damaged or absent fallopian tubes entirely. Unexplained infertility is thereby unique in the sense that pathology has not been found and so couples can technically rely on sexual intercourse alone to achieve pregnancy and not seek any active treatment. In reality, IVF is widely used in unexplained and mild male subfertility despite there being only a scarcity of evidence, particularly in the form of randomised trials, to support its widespread use in these instances [22, 23]. IVF should be a procedure for which careful consideration is taken in determining who should receive the treatment. The critical factor in terms of maximising the effective use of IVF in terms of live births appears to be the timing as to when the procedure should be recommended.

6.5.2.3 When Is the Right Time?

Timing of IVF use is a matter in which there is no real consensus. A randomised trial investigating different treatment strategies in unexplained infertility indicated that reducing number of IUI cycles with MOH such that IVF is commenced earlier leads to shorter time to pregnancy and cost reduction. However, there was a similar ongoing pregnancy rate in both randomised arms at 24 months [50]. Multiple pregnancy rates in the study were high in both arms.

Findings from several observational studies indicate that in couples with unexplained subfertility

Table 6.2 Comparison between sexual intercourse and first-line treatments in treatment of unexplained infertility

	Sexual intercourse vs. IUI	Sexual intercourse vs. IVF
Cochrane review summary	• Based on three RCTs • Total sample size = 690 • Live birth rates not significantly different in IUI (with or without COS) than sexual intercourse	• Based on two studies • Total sample size = 86 • Inadequate evidence to suggest IVF improves clinical pregnancy rates relative to sexual intercourse
Conclusions from the literature	• Benefit of IUI over sexual intercourse alone in couples with unexplained infertility is dependent on their prognosis for natural conception • IUI > sexual intercourse in poor prognosis, as seen by higher live birth rates in IUI after three cycles of each treatment • IUI = sexual intercourse in intermediate and good prognosis, as seen by comparable cumulative live birth rates in groups with 6 months of expectant management compared to immediate IUI groups	• Inconclusive evidence that IVF improves outcomes in treatment-naïve couples with unexplained infertility relative to sexual intercourse alone • Need for more robust studies to determine when to transition to IVF, as IVF is likely only to provide benefit over sexual intercourse in those that have a low chance of natural conception

COS, controlled ovarian stimulation; IUI, intrauterine insemination; IVF, in vitro fertilisation; RCT, randomised controlled trials.

waiting to undergo IVF, spontaneous conception occurs in a substantial proportion of couples who have had subfertility for a lower amount of time [51–53]. This was reflected in a nationwide cohort study conducted in the Netherlands, which found that the 12-month ongoing pregnancy rate was 15% in couples with unexplained infertility who were on the IVF waiting list [54].

Consideration of the preceding evidence supports the notion that early use of IVF in couples with unexplained subfertility, while able to promote conception, simply achieves the outcome of pregnancy faster than what would inevitably have happened through natural conception from a period of 6 months expectant management. Future studies should investigate how IVF compares to less invasive treatments in this population, taking into consideration prognostic indicators including the duration of infertility. Other studies, however, indicate no benefit from IVF over IUI in couples with unexplained infertility who start treatment, usually after 2 years of infertility [44].

6.5.2.4 How Safe Is IVF?

Discussion about IVF safety typically revolves around the high risk of developing (high order) multiple pregnancies, which itself has association with adverse maternal and perinatal outcomes [55]. Such complications include an increased maternal risk of developing gestational diabetes and pre-eclampsia and neonatal morbidity or mortality associated with an increased risk of premature delivery. There has been a well-embraced swing, by many in the field of IVF, towards performing elective SET as a means of reducing multiple pregnancy rate [56]. Despite this shift, transfers of more than one embryo still constitutes common practice in many regions of the world such as the United States and Asia, which still have high multiple birth rates of 20%–30% [57].

Although multiple pregnancy has a notable association with poor perinatal outcomes in IVF, it appears that mitigating this factor does not eliminate risk of adverse events entirely. Most children conceived from IVF are indeed born healthy; however, when compared with pregnancies that occur through natural conception, singleton IVF pregnancies have relatively poor obstetric and perinatal outcomes [55, 58–60]. Methods of embryo transfer used in IVF have also been implicated in different perinatal outcomes, with some studies showing worse perinatal outcomes following conception in fresh embryo transfer compared to frozen/thawed embryo; however, the data at this stage are inconclusive [61–63].

The use of extended embryo culture with single blastocyst transfer is another means put forth to circumvent risk of multiple pregnancy from IVF without compromising its high success rates per cycle; however, blastocyst transfer has been linked to higher rates of preterm birth and congenital malformations [64–66].

Concerns have been raised regarding the impact of IVF on the long-term health of children conceived through such means. Recent studies have demonstrated a correlation between IVF children who are generally 'healthy' but have higher rates of increased blood pressure, higher adiposity and blood sugar levels and greater generalised vascular dysfunction relative to those children born without medical intervention [67, 68]. These changes appear to be unrelated to parental subfertility but are seemingly attributable to the process of IVF itself. The reason for this could be related to epigenetic and developmental defects shown to occur in non-human mammal studies with IVF and other assisted reproductive technologies. There is a necessity for further verification of these potential complications of IVF through robust clinical studies, and so caution should be exercised until such time where there is a greater evidence base to draw firmer conclusions.

Synthesising the evidence put forth in the preceding text, the absolute risks of unfavourable outcomes in IVF seem to be acceptably low to justify offering it as treatment to couples with unexplained subfertility who have little likelihood of conceiving naturally. However, it is within reason to dispute subjecting couples to unnecessary risks if they have an otherwise reasonable prognosis. If the current trend of IVF use in infertility treatment continues, it is such that there will be an increasing number of couples with acceptable natural conception prognosis who unnecessarily undergo IVF and are consequently exposed to likely preventable risk of adverse outcomes.

If we conservatively estimate that 10% of the 4 million couples achieving pregnancy through IVF since 2003 could have delayed fertility treatment and trusted in natural conception or started with IUI or ovulation induction to achieve pregnancy, at least 400,000 couples therefore underwent IVF unnecessarily. From this, an estimation of the prevented adverse outcomes can be calculated. Considering a 20% twin rate, 80,000 twin pregnancies could have potentially been avoided, which in turn may have prevented 725 perinatal deaths in a developed country setting and adverse outcomes in another 2,500 children. Even if we applied IVF with SET instead of IVF DET in this same 400,000 theoretical cohort, the estimated additional adverse outcomes from IVF over other treatments might be 8,400 small-for-gestational age babies, 6,400 preterm births and 50 perinatal deaths.

6.6 Evidence-Based Recommendation

Considering what has been discussed thus far, it can be inferred that IUI and IVF are both therapies effective in the treatment of couples with unexplained infertility. Treatment efficacy, however, appears to be contingent on each individual couple's prognostic profile, whereby in couples with a good prognosis treatment does not confer added advantage. IUI notably appears to have limited benefit in couples with a poor natural conception prognosis. Therefore, before commencing IUI, each couple should have their chance of natural conception estimated with a prognostic predictive model. In couples with a good prognosis, IUI can be deferred in favour of expectant management coupled with tubal flushing and lifestyle modification. Couples with a poor natural conception prognosis, however, should progress directly to IUI.

IVF should be reserved for couples who have failed both expectant management and IUI. IVF, albeit seemingly more effective, has several associated downsides including increased OHSS and multiple pregnancy risk, among numerous other adverse maternal and fetal outcomes, and high financial cost. From an outcome perspective, namely in terms of successful pregnancy and financial considerations, adopting a more restrained approach to the treatment of unexplained infertility can enable provision of care through partial or complete economic reimbursements without compromising pregnancy outcomes. Figure 6.3 illustrates an evidence-based algorithm to approach treatment of couples with unexplained infertility.

The treatment flowchart progresses from left to right. Couples presenting for fertility assessment exhibit benefits to live birth rates following assessment of tubal patency using hysterosalpingography (HSG) with an oil-based contrast. Following an infertility work-up, a couple with unexplained infertility can have their prognosis for natural conception predicted using the validated Hunault synthesis model. Couples can be stratified into groups with either good prognosis (>30%) or poor prognosis (≤30%) for natural conception. Couples with good prognosis can trial 6 months of expectant management. Intrauterine insemination (IUI) with or without controlled ovarian stimulation (COS) for six cycles is indicated in those who fail 6 months of expectant management, and in those couples with an estimated poor prognosis for natural conception. First-line treatment should therefore be the more conservative options of expectant management and IUI. Failure of IUI with or without COS necessitates second-line treatment with assisted reproductive technology, including IVF or ICSI.

6.7 Conclusion

IVF has given many couples the opportunity of bearing children in instances in which they may have been

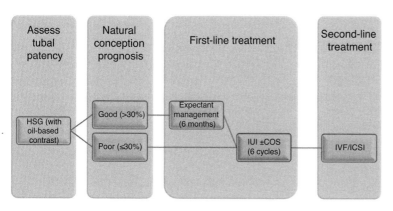

Figure 6.3 Evidence-based treatment algorithm for unexplained infertility.

unable to do so, proving itself to be a powerful instrument in treatment of infertility. Extending the use of IVF to instances outside of treatment of couples for whom spontaneous conception is unlikely or practically impossible is something that must be considered with care. Conditions in which the IVF efficacy is unverified, such as unexplained and mild male subfertility, warrant raising of the threshold before IVF is employed. As such, there exists an obligation of those in the field of IVF to the infertile and subfertile community to reserve IVF for those that require it, and to critically appraise any new evidence or innovations that arise. Indeed, one must strive to continually uphold among the most basic medical tenets – 'first, do no harm'.

References

1. Thoma ME, McLain AC, Louis JF, King RB, Trumble AC, Sundaram R, et al. Prevalence of infertility in the United States as estimated by the current duration approach and a traditional constructed approach. *Fertil Steril.* 2013;**99**(5):1324e31.e1321.

2. Te Velde ER, Eijkemans MJC, Habbema JDF. Variation in couple fecundity and time to pregnancy, an essential concept in human reproduction. *Lancet.* 2000;**355**:1928e9.

3. National Institute for Health and Care Excellence. Fertility: assessment and treatment for people with fertility problems. NICE Clinical Guideline; 2013. Available at: www.nice.org.uk/guidance/cg156/resourc es/%0Dupdated-niceguidelines-revise-treatment-recommendations-for-peoplewith-%0Dfertility-problems

4. Brandes M, Hamilton CJCM, de Bruin JP, Nelen WLDM, Kremer JAM. The relative contribution of IVF to the total ongoing pregnancy rate in a subfertile cohort. *Hum Reprod.* 2010;**25**(1):118e26.

5. ESHRE. Guidelines for counseling infertility. 2001.

6. Hunault CC, Habbema JDF, Eijkemans MJC, Collins JA, Evers JLH, te Velde ER. Two new prediction rules for spontaneous pregnancy leading to live birth among subfertile couples, based on the synthesis of three previous models. *Hum Reprod.* 2004;**19**:2019e26.

7. van der Steeg JW, Steures P, Eijkemans MJC, Habbema JDF, Hompes PGA, Broekmans FJ, et al. Pregnancy is predictable: a large-scale prospective external validation of the prediction of spontaneous pregnancy in subfertile couples. *Hum Reprod.* 2006;**22**:536e42.

8. Bostofte E, Bagger P, Michael A, Stakemann G. Fertility prognosis for infertile couples. *Fertil Steril.* 1993;**59**:102e7.

9. Snick HK, Snick TS, Evers JL, Collins JA. The spontaneous pregnancy prognosis in untreated subfertile couples: the Walcheren primary care study. *Hum Reprod.* 1997;**12**:1582e8.

10. Collins JA, Burrows EA, Wilan AR. The prognosis for live birth among untreated infertile couples. *Fertil Steril.* 1995;**64**: 22e8.

11. Eimers JM, te Velde ER, Gerritse R, Vogelzang ET, Looman CW, Habbema JDF. The prediction of the chance to conceive in subfertile couples. *Fertil Steril.* 1994;**61**:44e52.

12. Bahamondes L, Alma FA, Faundes A, Vera S. Score prognosis for the infertile couple based on historical factors and sperm analysis. *Int J Gynaecol Obstet.* 1994;**46**:311e5.

13. Wichmann L, Isola J, Tuohimaa P. Prognostic variables in predicting pregnancy: a prospective follow up study of 907 couples with an infertility problem. *Hum Reprod.* 1994;**9**:1102e8.

14. Bloomington MN. Institute for clinical systems improvement (ICSI). Diagnosis and management of basic infertility; 2004. Available at: www.guideline.gov/

15. Stolwijk AM, Zielhuis GA, Hamilton CJ, Straatman H, Hollanders JM, Goverde HJ, et al. Prognostic models for the probability of achieving an ongoing pregnancy after in-vitro fertilization and the importance of testing their predictive value. *Hum Reprod.* 1996;**11**:2298e303.

16. Wasson JH, Sox HC, Neff RK, Goldman L. Clinical prediction rules: applications and methodological standards. *N Engl J Med.* 1985;**313**:793e9.

17. Bleeker SE, Moll HA, Steyerberg EW, Donders AR, Derksen-Lubsen G, Grobbee DE, et al. External validation is necessary in prediction research: a clinical example. *J Clin Epidemiol.* 2003;**56**:826e32.

18. Bensdorp AJ, van der Steeg JW, Steures P, Habbema JDF, Hompes PGA, Bossuyt PMM, et al., CECERM Study Group. A revised prediction model for natural conception. *Reprod Biomed Online.* 2017;**34** (6):619e26.

19. Veltman-Verhulst SM, Hughes E, Ayeleke RO, Cohlen BJ. Intra-uterine insemination for unexplained subfertility. *Cochrane Database Syst Rev.* 2016;**2**: Cd001838.

20. Farquhar CM, Liu E, Armstrong S, Arroll N, Lensen S, Brown J. Intrauterine insemination with ovarian stimulation versus expectant management for unexplained infertility (TUI): a pragmatic, open-label, randomised, controlled, two-centre trial. *Lancet.* 2018;**391**:441e50.

21. van den Boogaard NM, Bensdorp AJ, Oude Rengerink K, Barnhart K, Bhattacharya S, Custers IM, et al. Prognostic profiles and the effectiveness of assisted conception: secondary analyses of

individual patient data. *Hum Reprod Update*. 2014; **20**(1):141–51.

22. Hughes EG, Beecroft ML, Wilkie V, Burville L, Claman P, Tummon I, et al. A multicentre randomized controlled trial of expectant management versus IVF in women with Fallopian tube patency. *Hum Reprod*. 2004;**19**:1105e9.

23. Pandian Z, Gibreel A, Bhattacharya S. In vitro fertilisation for unexplained subfertility. *Cochrane Database Syst Rev*. 2015: Cd003357.

24. Gnoth C, Godehardt D, Godehardt E, Frank-Herrmann P, Freundl G. Time to pregnancy: results of the German prospective study and impact on the management of infertility. *Hum Reprod*. 2003;**18**:1959e66.

25. Weir WC, Weir DR. Therapeutic value of salpingograms in infertility. *Fertil Steril*. 1951;**2**(6):514–22.

26. Johnson NP, Farquhar CM, Hadden WE, Suckling J, Yu Y, Sadler L. The FLUSH trial–flushing with lipiodol for unexplained (and endometriosis-related) subfertility by hysterosalpingography: a randomized trial. *Hum Reprod*. 2004;**19**(9):2043–51.

27. Nugent D, Watson AJ, Killick SR, Balen AH, Rutherford AJ. A randomized controlled trial of tubal flushing with lipiodol for unexplained infertility. *Fertil Steril*. 2002;**77**(1):173–5.

28. Ogata R, Nakamura G, Uchiumi Y, Yokoyamay M, Watanabe Y, Nozaki M, et al. Therapeutic efficacy of hysterosalpingography (HSG) in infertility, a prospective, randomized, clinical study. *Jpn J Fertil Steril*. 1993; **38**:91–94.

29. Mohiyiddeen L, Hardiman A, Fitzgerald C, Hughes E, Mol BWJ, Johnson N, et al. Tubal flushing for subfertility. *Cochrane Database Syst Rev*. 2015(**5**): CD003718.

30. Dreyer K, van Rijswijk J, Mijatovic V, Goddijn M, Verhoeve HR, van Rooij IAJ, et al. Oil-based or water-based contrast for hysterosalpingography in infertile women. *N Engl J Med*. 2017;**376**(21):2043–52.

31. Ramlau-Hansen CH, Thulstrup AM, Nohr EA, Bonde JP, Sørensen TI, Olsen J. Subfecundity in overweight and obese couples. *Hum Reprod*. 2007;**22**:1634–7.

32. van der Steeg JW, Steures P, Eijkemans MJ, Habbema JDF, Hompes PGA, Burggraaff JM, et al. Obesity affects spontaneous pregnancy chances in subfertile, ovulatory women. *Hum Reprod*. 2008;**23**:324–8.

33. Rich-Edwards JW, Goldman MB, Willett WC, Hunter DJ, Stampfer MJ, Colditz GA, et al. Adolescent body mass index and infertility caused by ovulatory disorder. *Am J Obstet Gynecol*. 1994;**171**:171–7.

34. Legro RS, Barnhart HX, Schlaff WD, Carr BR, Diamond MP, Carson SA, et al. Clomiphene, metformin, or both for infertility in the polycystic ovary syndrome. *N Engl J Med*. 2007;**356**:551–66.

35. Rittenberg V, Seshadri S, Sunkara SK, Sobaleva S, Oteng-Ntim E, El-Toukhy T. Effect of body mass index on IVF treatment outcome: an updated systematic review and meta-analysis. *Reprod Biomed Online*. 2011;**23**:421–39.

36. Practice Committee of the American Society for Reproductive Medicine. Obesity and reproduction: a committee opinion. *Fertil Steril*. 2015;**104**:1116–26.

37. National Institute for Clinical Excellence. *Fertility: assessment and treatment for people with fertility problems*. London: RCOG Press, 2004.

38. Mutsaerts MAQ, van Oers AM, Groen H, Burggraaff JM, Kuchenbecker WKH, Perquin DAM, et al. Randomized trial of a lifestyle program in obese infertile women. *N Engl J Med*. 2016;**374**(20):1942–53.

39. Kupka MS, D'Hooghe T, Ferraretti AP, de Mouzon J, Erb K, Castilla JA, et al. Assisted reproductive technology in Europe, 2011: results generated from European registers by ESHRE. *Hum Reprod*. 2016;**31**: dev319.

40. Goverde AJ, McDonnell J, Vermeiden JP, Schats R, Rutten FF, Schoemaker J. Intrauterine insemination or in-vitro fertilisation in idiopathic subfertility and male subfertility: a randomised trial and cost-effectiveness analysis. *Lancet*. 2000;**355**:13e8.

41. Custers IM, K€onig TE, Broekmans FJ, Hompes PGA, Kaaijk E, Oosterhuis J, et al. Couples with unexplained subfertility and unfavorable prognosis: a randomized pilot trial comparing the effectiveness of in vitro fertilization with elective single embryo transfer versus intrauterine insemination with controlled ovarian stimulation. *Fertil Steril*. 2011;**96**:1107e11011.e1.

42. Gameiro S, Boivin J, Peronace L, Verhaak CM. Why do patients discontinue fertility treatment? A systematic review of reasons and predictors of discontinuation in fertility treatment. *Hum Reprod Update*. 2012;**18**:652e69.

43. van Rumste MME, Custers IM, van Wely M, Koks CA, van Weering HGI, Beckers NGM, et al. IVF with planned single embryo transfer versus IUI with ovarian stimulation in couples with unexplained subfertility: an economic analysis. *Reprod Biomed Online*. 2014;**28**:336e42.

44. Bensdorp AJ, Tjon-Kon-Fat RI, Bossuyt PM, Koks CA, Oosterhuis GJ, Hoek A, et al. Prevention of multiple pregnancies in couples with unexplained or mild male subfertility: randomised controlled trial of in vitro fertilisation with single embryo transfer or in vitro fertilisation in modified natural cycle compared with

intrauterine insemination with controlled ovarian hyperstimulation. *BMJ*. 2015;**350**:g7771.

45. Tjon-Kon-Fat RI, Bensdorp AJ, Bossuyt PM, Koks C, Oosterhuis GJ, Hoek A, et al. Is IVF-served two different ways-more cost-effective than IUI with controlled ovarian hyperstimulation? *Hum Reprod*. 2015;**30**(10):2331e9.

46. Bahadur G, Homburg R, Muneer A, Racich P, Alangaden T, Al-Habib A, et al. First line fertility treatment strategies regarding IUI and IVF require clinical evidence. *Hum Reprod*. 2016;**31**:1141e6.

47. Deaton JL, Gibson M, Blackmer KM, Nakajima ST, Badger GJ, Brumsted JR. A randomized, controlled trial of clomiphene citrate and intrauterine insemination in couples with unexplained infertility or surgically corrected endometriosis. *Fertil Steril*. 1990;**54**:1083e8.

48. Steures P, van der Steeg JW, Hompes PG, Habbema JD, Eijkemans MJ, Broekmans FJ, et al. Collaborative effort on the clinical evaluation in reproductive medicine. Intrauterine insemination with controlled ovarian hyperstimulation versus expectant management for couples with unexplained subfertility and an intermediate prognosis: a randomised clinical trial. *Lancet*. 2006;**368**:216e21.

49. Bhattacharya S, Harrild K, Mollison J, Wordsworth S, Tay C, Harrold A, et al. Clomifene citrate or unstimulated intrauterine insemination compared with expectant management for unexplained infertility: pragmatic randomised controlled trial. *BMJ*. 2008;**337**:a716.

50. Reindollar RH, Regan MM, Neumann PJ, Levine BS, Thornton KL, Alper MM, et al. A randomized clinical trial to evaluate optimal treatment for unexplained infertility: the fast track and standard treatment (FASTT) trial. *Fertil Steril*. 2010;**94**:888e99.

51. Troude P, Bailly E, Guibert J, Bouyer J, de la Rochebrochard E, DAIFI Group. Spontaneous pregnancies among couples previously treated by in vitro fertilization. *Fertil Steril*. 2012;**98**:63e8.

52. van Dongen AJ, Verhagen TE, Dumoulin JC, Land JA, Evers JL. Reasons for dropping out from a waiting list for in vitro fertilization. *Fertil Steril*. 2010;**94**:1713e6.

53. Farquhar CM, van den Boogaard NM, Riddell C, Macdonald A, Chan E, Mol BW. Accessing fertility treatment in New Zealand: a comparison of the clinical priority access criteria with a prediction model for couples with unexplained subfertility. *Hum Reprod*. 2011;**26**:3037e44.

54. Eijkemans MJ, Lintsen AM, Hunault CC, Bouwmans CA, Hakkaart L, Braat DD, et al. Pregnancy chances on an IVF/ICSI waiting list: a national

prospective cohort study. *Hum Reprod*. 2008 Jul;**23** (7):1627e32.

55. Pandey S, Shetty A, Hamilton M, Bhattacharya S, Maheshwari A. Obstetric and perinatal outcomes in singleton pregnancies resulting from IVF/ICSI: a systematic review and meta-analysis. *Hum Reprod Update*. 2012;**18**:485e503.

56. Bergh C. Single embryo transfer: a mini-review. *Hum Reprod*. 2005;**2**:323e7.

57. ESHRE. ART (assisted reproductive technology) fact sheet. Internet site ESHRE. Available at: www.eshre.eu /annual_meeting/page.aspx/1367

58. Jackson RA, Gibson KA, Wu YW, Croughan MS. Perinatal outcomes in singletons following in vitro fertilization: a metaanalysis. *Obstet Gynecol*. 2004;**103**:551e63.

59. Helmerhorst FM, Perquin DAM, Donker D, Keirse MJNC. Perinatal outcome of singletons and twins after assisted conception: a systematic review of controlled studies. *BMJ*. 2004;**328**:261.

60. Barnhart KT. Assisted reproductive technologies and perinatal morbidity: interrogating the association. *Fertil Steril*. 2013; **99**:299e302.

61. Maheshwari A, Pandey S, Shetty A, Hamilton M, Bhattacharya S. Obstetric and Perinatal outcomes in singleton pregnancies resulting from the transfer of frozen thawed versus fresh embryos generated through in-vitro fertilisation treatment: a systematic review and meta-analysis. *Fertil Steril*. 2012;**98**:368e77.

62. Rumbold AR, Moore VM, Whitrow MJ, Oswald TK, Moran LJ, Fernandez RC, et al. The impact of specific fertility treatments on cognitive development in childhood and adolescence: a systematic review. *Hum Reprod*. 2017;**32**:1489e507.

63. Davies MJ, Rumbold AR, Marino JL, Willson K, Giles LC, Whitrow MJ, et al. Maternal factors and the risk of birth defects after IVF and ICSI: a whole of population cohort study. *BJOG*. 2017;**124**:1537e44.

64. Dar S, Librach CL, Gunby J, Bissonnette F, Cowan L, IVF Directors Group of Canadian Fertility and Andrology Society. Increased risk of preterm birth in singleton pregnancies after blastocyst versus Day 3 embryo transfer: Canadian ART Register (CARTR) analysis. *Hum Reprod*. 2013;**28**:924e8.

65. K€allen B, Finnstr€om O, Lindam A, Nilsson E, Nygren K-G, Olausson PO. Blastocyst versus cleavage stage transfer in in vitro fertilization: differences in neonatal outcome? *Fertil Steril*. 2010;**94**:1680e3.

66. Kansal Kalra S, Ratcliffe SJ, Barnhart KT, Coutifaris C. Extended embryo culture and an increased risk of preterm delivery. *Obstet Gynecol*. 2012;**120**:69e75.

67. Scherrer U, Rimoldi SF, Rexhaj E, Stuber T, Duplain H, Garcin S, et al. Systemic and pulmonary vascular

dysfunction in children conceived by assisted reproductive technologies. *Circulation*. 2012;**125** (15):1890e6.

68. Hart R, Norman RJ. The longer-term health outcomes for children born as a result of IVF treatment: Part I-General health outcomes. *Hum Reprod Update*. 2013;**19**:232e43.

Further Reading

Bensdorp AJ, van der Steeg JW, Steures P, Habbema JDF, Hompes PGA, Bossuyt PMM, et al., CECERM Study Group. A revised prediction model for natural conception. *Reprod Biomed Online*. 2017 Jun;**34**(6):619e26.

Farquhar CM, Liu E, Armstrong S, Arroll N, Lensen S, Brown J. Intrauterine insemination with ovarian stimulation versus expectant management for unexplained infertility (TUI): a pragmatic, open-label, randomised, controlled, two-centre trial. *Lancet*. 2018;**391**:441e50.

Goverde AJ, McDonnell J, Vermeiden JP, Schats R, Rutten FF, Schoemaker J. Intrauterine insemination or in-vitro fertilisation in idiopathic subfertility and male subfertility: a randomised trial and cost-effectiveness analysis. *Lancet*. 2000;**355**:13e8.

Hughes EG, Beecroft ML, Wilkie V, Burville L, Claman P, Tummon I, et al. A multicentre randomized controlled trial of expectant management versus IVF in women with Fallopian tube patency. *Hum Reprod*. 2004;**19**:1105e9.

Pandey S, Shetty A, Hamilton M, Bhattacharya S, Maheshwari A. Obstetric and perinatal outcomes in singleton pregnancies resulting from IVF/ICSI: a systematic review and meta-analysis. *Hum Reprod Update*. 2012;**18**:485e503.

Reindollar RH, Regan MM, Neumann PJ, Levine BS, Thornton KL, Alper MM, et al. A randomized clinical trial to evaluate optimal treatment for unexplained infertility: the fast track and standard treatment (FASTT) trial. *Fertil Steril*. 2010;**94**: 888e99.

van der Steeg JW, Steures P, Eijkemans MJC, Habbema JDF, Hompes PGA, Broekmans FJ, et al. Pregnancy is predictable: a large-scale prospective external validation of the prediction of spontaneous pregnancy in subfertile couples. *Hum Reprod*. 2006;**22**:536e42.

Veltman-Verhulst SM, Hughes E, Ayeleke RO, Cohlen BJ. Intra-uterine insemination for unexplained subfertility. *Cochrane Database Syst Rev*. 2016;**2**:Cd001838.

Assisted Reproduction
Role in the Management of Infertility

Kugajeevan Vigneswaran and Haitham Hamoda

7.1 Introduction

Assisted reproduction technology (ART) encompasses fertility treatments which require manipulation of oocyte, sperm or both in vitro. This chapter aims to provide an overview of ART, including indications for treatment as well as the procedures involved. This will also include complications of ART as well as the evidence assessing the perinatal outcomes of children resulting from ART.

Techniques uses in assisted reproduction include the following:

- Intrauterine insemination
- In vitro fertilization/intracytoplasmic sperm injection
- Gamete intrafallopian transfer/zygote intrafallopian transfer
- Oocyte donation
- Surrogacy

7.2 Intrauterine Insemination (with or without Ovarian Stimulation)

Intrauterine insemination (IUI) describes the placement of prepared sperm into the uterine cavity around the time of ovulation. This can be done within a natural menstrual cycle or in combination with ovarian stimulation. The latter is used to induce ovulation in anovulatory women but can also be carried out in women with ovulatory cycles, with the rationale of increasing the number of eggs available for fertilisation.

John Hunter is credited with the first documented IUI procedure in the 1770s, when he advised a man with hypospadias to inject his seminal fluid using a syringe into his wife's vagina, and this resulted in a pregnancy.

IUI is generally used when there are patent fallopian tubes and normal sperm parameters. The rationale for the use of IUI is to increase the density of motile sperm available for fertilisation of the oocyte. Preparation of the sperm removes dead and immotile sperms as well as debris, white cells and seminal plasma, which can interfere with fertilisation. IUI also bypasses the cervix, thus potentially avoiding cervical mucus problems.

7.2.1 Indications for IUI

The National Institute for Health and Care Excellence (NICE) fertility guidelines in 2013 [1] outlined several indications for which IUI could be considered. These included couples for whom vaginal sexual intercourse would be difficult, such as those where one partner has a physical disability or psychosexual problems. Other indications for IUI include the use of donor sperm in women in same-sex relationships and scenarios that require sperm washing such as HIV-positive men to minimise the risk of viral transmission.

The NICE fertility guidelines recommended that IUI should not be routinely offered in cases of unexplained infertility, mild endometriosis or mild male factor infertility, where regular unprotected intercourse was possible. This recommendation was based on randomised controlled trial (RCT) data from two studies comparing expectant management with both natural cycle IUI as well as stimulated cycle IUI (with gonadotropin therapy). One of these studies, by Bhattacharya et al. in 2008, was a three-arm study that included 580 women and concluded that there was no significant advantage to be gained with IUI over expectant management in relation to the primary outcome, namely live birth rates [2].

The NICE fertility guidelines 2013 literature review concluded that low-quality evidence comparing IUI with stimulation and IUI without stimulation did show a significantly higher live birth rate with stimulation. However, this was accompanied by a higher multiple pregnancy rate. The guideline group concluded that IVF provided greater control in regard to the number of embryos transferred and felt that several cycles of IUI with stimulation would be required to match the live birth rates achieved with a single cycle of IVF.

The NICE guideline recommendations led to a decline in the number of IUI cycles performed, with the Human Fertilisation & Embryology Authority (HFEA) data report in 2018 indicating a 50% decrease in the total number of procedures since 2013 [3].

In 2018, results from a pragmatic RCT were published designed to evaluate the use of IUI with ovarian stimulation for couples with unexplained infertility [4].

The trial randomised 201 women with unexplained infertility to either having three cycles of IUI with clomiphene citrate or letrozole or three cycles of expectant management. The former was associated with a three-fold greater live birth rate than the latter (31% vs. 9%), with a relatively low multiple pregnancy rate. The data were analysed on an intention to treat basis and it was of note that nearly 25% of the pregnancies in the IUI arm arose naturally, that is, independent of the intervention.

The group concluded that IUI with ovarian stimulation was a safe and effective treatment for couples with unexplained infertility and an unfavourable prognosis for natural conception.

Overall success rates with IUI will vary and are largely dependent on female age as well as the quality of injected sperm. Guidelines indicate that the concentration of progressively motile sperm is the most predictive factor for chance of success with IUI and generally recommend a cut-off of at least 5 million sperm being inseminated to optimise outcomes.

National UK data from 2016 showed an overall birth rate of 12% per treatment cycle of IUI. The highest success rates were observed in women less than 38 years of age (14% in women less than 35 years of age and 12% for women 35–37 years old). Beyond the age of 42 years, the live birth rates were low. The multiple pregnancy rates were recorded as 8%.

In summary, IUI is an effective and safe treatment option for patients who are unable to have regular vaginal sexual intercourse. The evidence suggests that in the context of unexplained infertility, IUI without ovarian stimulation does not appear to offer a significant advantage over expectant management. However, when combined with ovarian stimulation, there may be an improvement in live birth rates compared to expectant management alone.

IUI with ovarian stimulation provides a less invasive treatment option when compared with IVF, although the latter is likely to be more successful. Further research is required to compare the efficacy of cumulative cycles of IUI compared to IVF. IUI combined with ovarian stimulation may therefore offer an option in unexplained infertility, particularly for younger women who are not yet ready to proceed with IVF.

7.2.2 Monitoring

To ascertain the optimal timing of the insemination procedure as well as to ensure safety where stimulation has been carried out, monitoring of folliculogenesis by transvaginal pelvic ultrasound is utilised. Typically, serial ultrasound scans from day 10 of the menstrual cycle are performed to allow assessment of the number and size of dominant follicles. In cycles where more than two stimulated follicles have been detected on tracking, cancellation of the IUI cycle should be advised because of the higher risk of multiple pregnancies. The couple should be advised in this situation to avoid unprotected intercourse.

Monitoring of a luteinising hormone (LH) surge is also undertaken to determine the optimal time for insemination. IUIs are typically carried out within 24 hours of the LH surge as assessed by urinary ovulation prediction kits. Alternatively, ovulation can be triggered by the administration of human chorionic gonadotropin (hCG) once the leading follicle is 16–18 mm diameter followed by insemination approximately 36 hours later.

7.2.3 Procedure

Fresh semen is produced by masturbation after approximately 2–7 days of abstinence. The sperm is then prepared and drawn up in a catheter, passed gently through the cervical canal and injected into the uterine cavity.

7.2.4 Complications

The main complication of IUI is multiple pregnancy associated with ovarian stimulation. There is a small risk of developing ovarian hyperstimulation syndrome (OHSS) in cycles stimulated with gonadotropins. The risk of ectopic pregnancy or miscarriage has not been shown to increase in IUI cycles compared with natural conceptions. The reported risk of pelvic inflammatory disease after IUI has been estimated at 0.01%–0.2%.

7.3 In Vitro Fertilisation

The development of IVF has revolutionised the management of infertile couples and since the birth of Louise Brown in 1978, it is estimated that more than 8 million children have been born from IVF. Live birth rates with IVF have steadily increased over the years largely as a result of clinical improvements and advances in laboratory technology and expertise.

7.3.1 Ovarian Stimulation

Early cycles of IVF performed by Edwards and Steptoe required the retrieval of a mature oocyte during a natural cycle for patients with fallopian tube defects. IVF has since found a wider application in the management of other causes of infertility including male factor, anovulation as well as unexplained infertility. Ovarian stimulation prior to oocyte retrieval became standard practice with the objective of increasing the number of oocytes collected and consequently increasing the pool of embryos available to select from for transfer.

Ovarian reserve tests serve to counsel IVF patients and guide clinicians in predicting the likely ovarian response to stimulation. Using a combination of antral follicle count and anti-mullerian hormone assessment along with female age, it is possible to estimate oocyte numbers at retrieval thereby optimising ovarian stimulation in IVF.

7.3.1.1 Pituitary Control

In the early years following its introduction, IVF was carried out using gonadotropins for controlled ovarian stimulation, but without pituitary suppression. This resulted in less flexibility with both the scheduling of IVF cycles and the timing of oocyte retrievals, which resulted in collections being performed at night and throughout weekends. This also resulted in higher cycle cancellation rates owing to the frequent occurrence of a premature endogenous LH surge prior to oocyte retrieval.

The introduction of gonadotropin-releasing hormone (GnRH) *agonists* for pituitary suppression in the mid-1980s to be used alongside gonadotropin ovarian stimulation enabled greater planning of controlled ovarian stimulation. Once downregulation had been achieved, oocyte retrieval could be timed to precisely 34–38 hours following administration of hCG, which serves as a surrogate for the mid-cycle LH surge and causes resumption of meiosis within an oocyte, in preparation for fertilisation.

GnRH agonists can be administered using intranasal, subcutaneous or intramuscular preparations. There are several proposed regimens when using GnRH agonist therapy for pituitary downregulation. In the *long GnRH agonist protocol,* the agonist is commenced in the mid-luteal phase of the preceding cycle before commencing ovarian stimulation, resulting in a 10–14-day lead-in to treatment. The objective of this is to allow time for the initial 'flare effect' that GnRH agonist administration will have on the pituitary gland to wear off before pituitary desensitisation is achieved 8–10 days later. Once pituitary downregulation has been achieved, stimulation with gonadotropins can begin. Downregulation can be confirmed by ultrasound (thin endometrium and quiescent ovaries), and this will be associated with low serum follicle stimulating hormone FSH, LH and oestradiol levels. The *short GnRH agonist protocol* involves commencing the agonist in the early follicular phase of the IVF cycle to take advantage of the initial flare effect on the pituitary gland before desensitisation is achieved. The *ultrashort protocol,* on the other hand, involves administering GnRH agonist for only 2–3 days in the early follicular phase using only the flare-up effect, with some studies reporting its use in poor responders.

The literature suggests comparable efficacy between the long and short GnRH agonist protocols for pituitary suppression with IVF, although there is limited evidence assessing the role of the ultrashort GnRH agonist protocol in this context. In practice, the long protocol remains the most commonly used GnRH agonist regimen.

In 1994, *GnRH antagonists* were introduced as an additional option to GnRH agonists in preventing premature LH surges in controlled ovarian stimulation. The GnRH antagonist acts immediately on the pituitary and prevents pituitary secretion of both FSH and LH, without the need for desensitisation. Ovarian stimulation could begin on day 2 of the menstrual cycle and daily administration of the antagonist would typically begin on day 5 or 6 of stimulation or once the leading follicle had reached 14 mm (usually by day 6–7). A fixed start (beginning on day 5 or 6 of stimulation) protocol seems to be comparable in regard to clinical outcomes when compared with a flexible start (once the leading follicle had reached 14 mm) protocol.

By eliminating the need for pituitary desensitisation, antagonist cycles are much shorter and more convenient for patients and have been shown to require lower total gonadotropin doses. Furthermore, there appears to be a reduced risk of OHSS. In antagonist cycles this risk reducing advantage is furthered by the discovery that the final maturation of oocytes can be initiated by using a single dose of GnRH agonist instead of hCG. The LH rise induced with an agonist trigger has a shorter half-life than that of hCG and this reduces the OHSS risk significantly.

A recently updated meta-analysis including all RCTs to date comparing GnRH agonist versus antagonist regimes revealed similar IVF success rates, with a lower overall consumption of gonadotropins and a reduced risk of OHSS with antagonist cycles [5].

The combined contraceptive pill (COCP) has been commonly used as pretreatment with IVF. This allows greater control with the scheduling of IVF cycles and may prevent the development of ovarian cysts which can occur with the flare effect of starting treatment with a GnRH agonist. A recent meta-analysis, however, showed a slight reduction in clinical pregnancy rates with the COCP (risk ratio [RR] 0.80, 95% confidence interval [CI] 0.66–0.97).

7.3.1.2 Gonadotropins

Human pituitary gonadotropins were first extracted in 1958, from cadaveric human pituitaries. In 1954, it had also been discovered that FSH and LH could be extracted from the urine of post-menopausal women. Human menopausal gonadotropin (hMG) was proposed for therapy in humans in 1957. The initial products required very large volumes of urine (3.5 L required per 75 IU of FSH) and contained several other unwanted urinary proteins. In the absence of an alternative, hMG was used to induce ovulation in hypogonadotropic patients as well as anovulatory normogonadotrophic patients.

In the early 1980s hMG/hCG protocols became standard practice for assisted reproduction cycles, shifting from monofollicular development to super-ovulation with multiple follicles (Figure 7.1).

Highly purified hMG followed in 2004, which was produced through an eight-step purification process of menopausal urine. Part of this process incorporated immunological techniques and utilised specific monoclonal antibodies to FSH and LH. Following these steps, hypersensitivity was minimised and consequently it was possible to produce a subcutaneous preparation for injection.

Recombinant human FSH (rFSH) was developed to eliminate the inherent variation found with urinary FSH products as well as ensuring greater availability of a product not reliant on urinary donation. The

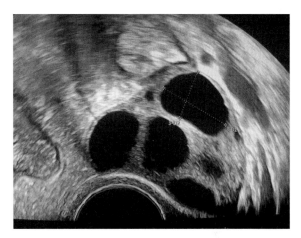

Figure 7.1 Ultrasound image of a stimulated ovary showing multiple follicles.

increased purity of rFSH reduced the possibility of oxidation and led to the production of liquid gonadotropin formulations, dispensed in prefilled injection devices.

Systematic review and meta-analysis data suggested that adding recombinant human LH (rLH) to rFSH for ovarian stimulation may improve pregnancy outcomes in poor responders compared with rFSH alone. Subsequently, however, an RCT (ESPART 2016) assessed this question in poor responders and included 462 women randomised to IVF with rFSH/rLH and 477 to IVF with rFSH alone. The study found no significant difference in the number of oocytes retrieved between the two groups.

In summary, current evidence which includes an updated Cochrane review shows similar efficacy between urinary and recombinant gonadotropins including the use of FSH alone or combined FSH/LH preparations with respect to implantation rates, live births and multiple pregnancy rates.

7.3.1.3 FSH Dose

The starting dose of gonadotropins used in IVF is typically between 150 and 300 IU of FSH, with the treatment dose often based on the patient's age and her ovarian reserve. Patients at risk of developing OHSS can be started on relatively low doses of 100–150 IU per day. Lower doses of 75 IU per day do not appear to be sufficient for most women.

An RCT (OPTIMIST) reported no clinically significant difference in cumulative live birth rates when using individualised FSH dosing regimens (100–450 IU) compared to a standard dose regimen (150 IU). The study, however, noted significantly higher cancellation rates and significantly higher rates of OHSS in the standard dose arm compared to the individualised arm. Several limitations need to be considered when interpreting the data reported in the OPTIMIST trial including that adjustments in FSH doses were allowed in the standard dose arm after the first cycle and cumulative outcomes were assessed only up to 18 months.

A Cochrane review published in 2018 concluded that tailoring the FSH dose in any particular population (low, normal, high ovarian reserve), did not appear to influence the rates of live birth/ongoing pregnancy. The review, however, concluded that individualisation of FSH doses reduced the overall incidence of moderate and severe OHSS. The authors noted that there were sample size limitations in the studies included that need to be considered when interpreting these data [6].

In summary, evidence from recent randomised studies suggests that the concept of individualised FSH dosing in IVF may not necessarily offer a significant advantage in terms of live births with IVF but does appear to reduce the risk of OHSS and lowers the risk of cycle cancellation. There are limitations to the methodology and study sample size of these reports which suggest one should exercise caution in the interpretation of these findings. More research is needed to evaluate this further.

7.3.1.4 Poor Responders

A description of poor response to fertility treatment was first defined by Garcia in 1983 as peak oestradiol levels of less than 300 pg/mL following controlled ovarian stimulation with 150 IU of hMG.

The European Society of Human Reproduction (ESHRE) provided a more recent definition of poor ovarian response (Bologna criteria 2011) as having at least two of the following three features:

- Advanced maternal age >40 or other factors for diminished ovarian reserve
- Previous history of poor ovarian response (fewer than three oocytes retrieved with conventional ovarian stimulation)
- An abnormal ovarian reserve test (AFC <5–7 follicles or AMH <5.4 pmol/L)

IVF treatment for patients with diminished ovarian reserve can be challenging and is often associated with poor clinical outcomes, namely high risk of cycle cancellation and low pregnancy rates.

There is no consensus on what constitutes the optimal stimulation protocol for poor responders, although it is common practice to use high-dose FSH in such cycles. Some studies have reported on using low doses of FSH for ovarian stimulation or no FSH (natural cycle IVF) in such cases, instead of using high-dose FSH for ovarian stimulation. There is limited published evidence to guide practice and further research is required to assess the optimal treatment regimen in this context.

7.3.1.5 Monitoring During IVF

Monitoring ovarian response to superovulation is usually performed using vaginal ultrasound tracking of the follicular response to stimulation. Approximately from day 8–10 of stimulation, measurement of the number and average diameter of each follicle within the ovaries is calculated, typically on alternate days, with stimulated follicles expected to grow by 2 mm a day. Endometrial thickness is also noted during these scans. The pre-ovulatory hCG trigger can be administered once a set number of leading follicles reaches at least 17 mm (many clinical protocols aim for at least 3) and a satisfactory cohort of intermediate follicles has been achieved.

The use of biochemical indicators of follicular activity, namely serum oestradiol concentrations, may aid clinical decision-making in women at risk of OHSS although they appear of limited clinical value in women with normal or low ovarian reserve. A Cochrane review (2014) concluded that there was no evidence to suggest that combined monitoring by transvaginal pelvic ultrasound scan and serum oestradiol is more efficacious than monitoring by transvaginal pelvic ultrasound scan alone in respect of clinical pregnancy rates or the incidence of OHSS. However, the quality of the evidence assessing this was noted to be low. The authors concluded that a combined monitoring protocol including both transvaginal pelvic ultrasound scan and serum oestradiol would be precautionary good clinical practice in a subset of women considered at high risk of OHSS.

7.3.2 Oocyte Retrieval

In the early to mid-1980s transvaginal ultrasound guided oocyte retrieval was introduced into IVF practice, allowing a move away from laparoscopic oocyte retrieval which necessitated the use of general anaesthesia in hospital and a more invasive surgical procedure.

A Danish group reported the first ultrasound-guided oocyte retrieval in 1981. For the initial few years, this was performed with transabdominal ultrasound, utilising a full urinary bladder as an acoustic window to perform transabdominal puncture of mature ovarian follicles. By 1983, transvaginal ultrasound was developed to allow for transvaginal oocyte retrieval using a para-cervical block for local anaesthesia.

Transvaginal ultrasound guided follicle aspiration is now the gold standard for oocyte retrieval. NICE guidelines endorse the use of conscious sedation as a safe and acceptable method of analgesia. The administration of sedatives must be performed in a way that adheres to safe practice guidelines and can include a combination of benzodiazepines, midazolam, opiates and occasionally propofol. Local anaesthetic can also be injected into the vaginal fornices for additional analgesia.

A clinicians' survey conducted in the United Kingdom in 2003 reported that 84% of units used intravenous sedation while the remaining 16% used general anaesthesia.

Follicle flushing refers to the process of refilling an aspirated follicle with culture medium and aspirating again in an attempt to dislodge an oocyte that is adherent to the follicular wall.

A recent systematic review which included three RCTS encompassing a total of 210 patients, comparing follicular flushing with no flushing found no benefit in any of the outcomes studied with flushing. NICE have suggested that follicle flushing may be beneficial in women with a very low number of follicles (two or less). There is limited evidence assessing the role of follicular flushing in women with low ovarian reserve, and further research is required to assess this.

The rate of severe complications with oocyte retrieval is very low and has been estimated at 0.08%, in a study numbering 7,000 IVF cycles. These may include vascular or visceral injury (0.2%), pelvic infection (0.4%) and adnexal torsion (0.1%).

7.3.3 Laboratory Procedures

The steps involved with insemination of the retrieved oocytes including ICSI, embryo culture and details on the techniques involved in cryopreservation are dealt with in Chapter 9.

7.3.4 Embryo Transfer

The objective of the embryo transfer procedure is to place the embryo(s) in the uppermiddle part of the endometrial cavity and to carry out the procedure with minimal endometrial trauma. The latter may induce uterine contractility and lower the chances of successful implantation. The American Society for Reproductive Medicine Committee guidelines recommend an upper or mid-cavity transfer with the embryo placed at least 10 mm away from the fundus.

7.3.4.1 Ultrasound

The use of ultrasound to guide the introduction of the embryo transfer catheter can overcome difficulties related to distorted anatomy of the cervical canal and uterus and may minimise the risk of endometrial trauma.

A recent meta-analysis included 14 RCTs and reported an improvement in clinical pregnancy and live birth rates with transabdominal ultrasound guidance during embryo transfer compared with conventional 'clinical touch'. No significant difference was noted in miscarriage and ectopic pregnancy rates. Transabdominal and transvaginal ultrasound have been shown to have equal efficacy.

7.3.4.2 Type of Embryo Transfer Catheter

Several catheters are available for the loading and placement of embryos into the uterine cavity. Soft catheters can follow the contours of the endometrial cavity and as a result can minimise endometrial trauma. In cases of cervical stenosis or uterine distortion, a stiff catheter may be required to facilitate the introduction of the embryo transfer catheter into the uterine cavity. Published evidence does not suggest a significant difference in implantation or pregnancy rates between the different catheters.

7.3.4.3 Technique

Care should be taken to inject the fluid containing the embryo slowly into the endometrial cavity. This is based on work performed on mouse embryos, which showed a rapidly injected embryo was more likely to collapse and undergo apoptosis when compared to slowly injected embryos. It is also important that time between loading the embryo into the catheter and transfer should be minimised to reduce environmental stress on the embryo once it leaves the incubator.

There are two main techniques employed for the placement of embryos within the uterine cavity:

1. Two-stage technique

   a. Initial placement of the outer catheter within the cervical canal up to the level or just beyond the internal os.

   b. Loading of inner catheter with embryo(s) and placement through the outer catheter under ultrasound guidance within the uterus below the fundus.

2. One-stage technique

   a. The inner catheter is loaded with the embryo(s) and the inner and outer catheter are passed to the embryo transfer practitioner as a single unit.

   b. The inner/outer single unit is then threaded through the external os/cervical canal and into the uterus to the desired level.

Both techniques are commonly used, although the two-stage method allows the embryos to remain in the incubator for as long as possible and they are removed only when there is 'certainty' of an uncomplicated transfer.

Fluid volumes used within the inner catheter for loading embryos are the same for both methods, typically 30 μL.

Bed rest post procedure has not been shown to be advantageous, with a number of RCTs showing no beneficial effect with bed rest after the embryo transfer procedure.

Sometimes a trial transfer is conducted before the IVF cycle start. This may be considered in cases where there is a perceived risk of a difficult transfer ahead, for example, previous cervical surgery fixed retroverted uterus, fibroids, uterine abnormality. If a problem is encountered at the trial transfer then cervical dilatation may be recommended before the cycle of ovarian stimulation commences.

7.3.4.4 Cleavage Stage or Blastocyst Transfer

Improvements in the laboratory conditions and culture media has enabled the reliable culture of embryos to the blastocyst stage (day 5–6). This may allow better selection of embryos for transfer or cryopreservation.

A Cochrane review included data from RCTs conducted up until April 2016, comprising a total of 4,031 women from 27 trials showed higher clinical pregnancy rates and live birth rates with fresh blastocyst transfers compared with fresh cleavage stage embryo transfers. This equated to 29% of women achieving a live birth after a fresh cleavage transfer, compared to between 32% and 42% after a fresh blastocyst transfer.

7.3.4.5 Number of Transferred Embryos

The decision regarding the number of embryos to transfer in an IVF cycle is often centred around a balance between increasing the chances of achieving a pregnancy yet minimising the risk of multiple pregnancy. The multiple pregnancy rate with IVF predominantly relates to the number of embryos replaced. In the early years of IVF it was common practice to transfer more than one embryo, and as a result IVF often resulted in multiple pregnancies with all their related adverse effects to mother and baby. The health implications of multiple pregnancy to mother and baby are discussed in more detail in Section 7.3.8.2.

The HFEA Code of Practice (9th edition) states that women under the age of 40 should not have more than two embryos replaced in any treatment cycle and those aged 40 or over should have no more than three embryos replaced. In a drive to reduce multiple pregnancy rates, the HFEA launched its 'One at a Time' campaign in 2007. The objective of this was to encourage a policy of single embryo replacement and set targets for clinics in the United Kingdom to reduce their multiple pregnancy rates to 10%. This resulted in a reduction in the multiple pregnancy rates from 24% in 2008 to 11% in 2016.

The single-embryo strategy was also endorsed by the NICE fertility guidelines (2013) promoting the concept of transferring a single fresh embryo and freezing any surplus embryos for subsequent transfer if the fresh transfer is unsuccessful. In addition, the NICE guidelines (2013) considered that extension of embryo culture to the blastocyst stage (day 5) instead of the then conventional cleavage stage (day 2–3) transfer would allow better selection of embryos and thus further encourage a policy of elective single-embryo transfer. The NICE guidelines promoted this by recommending the following:

- A single-embryo transfer for women under the age of 37
- A single-embryo transfer when a good quality embryo is available for women aged 37–39
- For women aged 40–42 consider double-embryo transfer

The NICE fertility guidelines also recommended a single-embryo transfer (at any age) where a good quality blastocyst is available and not to transfer more than two embryos during any one IVF cycle.

7.3.5 Luteal Phase Support

7.3.5.1 Physiological Basis for Luteal Support

The luteal phase is defined as the period between ovulation and either the establishment of a pregnancy or the onset of menses 2 weeks later.

Following ovulation, hormonal secretions from the corpus luteum result in secretory transformation of the endometrium. When pregnancy occurs, the formation and subsequent implantation of a blastocyst, the uterus becomes a source of hCG, which maintains the corpus luteum, owing to its similarity to LH and its ability to stimulate the same receptors as LH.

Implantation relies on the endometrium becoming receptive under the influence of progesterone secreted by the corpus luteum. During the luteal phase, there is a window of implantation that opens, at which point the embryo undergoes apposition, adherence and finally invasion of the endometrium. This is thought to occur between days 22 and 24 of a 28-day menstrual cycle.

The luteal phase of almost all IVF cycles is defective, and this is likely to be multifactorial in aetiology. Plausible explanations include disruption of follicular granulosa cells during oocyte retrieval, leading to suboptimal progesterone synthesis from the remnants of the corpora lutea. The impact of GnRH agonist downregulation is also thought to result in delayed recovery of pituitary function. However, a deficient luteal phase has also been observed with GnRH antagonist IVF cycles with compromised chances for pregnancy if no additional luteal support is given.

In addition, supraphysiological levels of steroids secreted by the numerous corpora lutea in the early luteal phase, and the subsequent suppression of LH release at the hypothalamic–pituitary axis via negative feedback mechanisms are likely to play a role in this process as well with LH withdrawal causing premature luteolysis.

To counter this deficiency in the luteal phase of IVF cycles, luteal phase support in the form of progesterone is recommended. Exogenous progesterone can be administered using oral, vaginal, rectal, subcutaneous (SC) or intramuscular (IM) preparations. Parenteral progesterone therapy has become the mainstay of treatment, as oral formulations undergo first pass liver metabolism and may result in poorly sustained plasma concentrations. IM progesterone needs to be given daily and is limited by pain as well as local site reactions. The SC route, on the other hand, is relatively well tolerated and has been shown to be as efficient as vaginal preparations.

Vaginal progesterone has become a first-line method of luteal phase support. Peak plasma concentrations are achieved at 3–8 hours, with a fall in levels over the next 8 hours. Therefore, daily doses of between 300 and 600 mg of vaginal progesterone are given, divided into two or three doses. There is thought to be a local mode of action within the endometrium and myometrium with vaginally administered progesterone, prior to entry into the systemic circulation. In the event of vaginal irritation and discharge causing discomfort, rectal administration can be considered.

7.3.5.2 Timing and Duration of Luteal Phase Support

As the window of receptivity within the endometrium is steroid dependent, supplementation must commence only after ovulation. Therefore, the start time for progesterone is generally recommended to be the night of oocyte retrieval in hCG-triggered cycles.

Once a pregnancy has established, the embryo is capable of releasing hCG, which compensates for the deficiency of endogenous LH. There is a wide variation in practice with respect to duration of progesterone administration. A meta-analysis to ascertain optimal duration of supplementation following IVF found that beyond the first positive hCG test, exogenous progesterone is unlikely to be necessary; however, there is a need for large randomised trials to assess this further.

7.3.6 Cryopreservation of Embryos

The objective of embryo cryopreservation is to retain morphologically normal surplus embryos not transferred in a fresh cycle to be utilised within a subsequent frozen embryo replacement cycle, thereby increasing the cumulative chances of pregnancy per oocyte retrieval performed. The first pregnancy resulting from a frozen human embryo occurred in 1985, and since then there has been a dramatic rise in the number of frozen embryo replacement cycles.

Embryos are stored in liquid nitrogen at −196°C, at either the early cleavage stages (days 2–3) or the blastocyst stage (day 5–6). Conventionally, this has been achieved using a slow freezing technique with low concentrations of cryoprotectants to avoid ice crystal formation. In recent years, rapid freezing using vitrification with higher concentrations of cryoprotectants has been used. Vitrification has resulted in a significant improvement in the success rates of frozen embryo replacement cycles as well as that of cryopreserved oocytes.

Many studies on pregnancy and live birth rates using vitrification show similar levels of success to those with fresh embryos and higher than those noted with slow freezing techniques. Vitrification has now largely superseded slow freezing as the method of choice for cryopreserving embryos as well as oocytes and ovarian tissue. A number of recent RCTs have suggested that elective freezing of all embryos in a fresh IVF cycle followed by frozen embryo transfer in subsequent cycles may improve pregnancy rates. A recent large multicentre RCT in China involving infertile women with polycystic ovary syndrome (PCOS) undergoing IVF showed that those who received frozen embryos had a significantly higher rate of live birth than did those receiving fresh embryos (49% vs. 42%, $P = 0.004$) as well as a lower risk of developing OHSS [7]. A parallel RCT assessing the same concept in women without PCOS included a total of 782 women and showed no significant difference in the rate of ongoing pregnancy or live birth between frozen-embryo transfer and fresh-embryo transfer in women without PCOS who were undergoing IVF.

A more recent meta-analysis included 11 studies with a total of 5,379 patients and reported a significant increase in live birth rates with elective frozen embryo replacement compared with fresh embryo transfer in hyper-responders but no differences were noted in live birth rates in normal responders. The risk of OHSS, however, was significantly lower with frozen embryo replacement in both hyper-responders and normo-responders [8].

Currently, a multicentre RCT (E-FREEZE) is underway in the United Kingdom to address the same question, assessing this both in women with and without PCOS. Replacement of frozen embryos can be carried out within a spontaneous natural menstrual cycle or within a hormone replacement cycle. The former requires the patient to have regular menstrual cycles and involves monitoring follicular development with serial ultrasound scans and identification of the endogenous LH surge. Once the latter is detected, the embryo transfer will be scheduled, usually 4 days later for a cryopreserved cleavage stage embryo and 6 days later for a cryopreserved blastocyst.

When embryo replacement is carried out within a hormone replacement cycle the endometrium is stimulated with oestrogen supplementation in the form of tablets or transdermal preparations (patches or gel) to induce endometrial proliferation. Once adequate endometrial thickness is detected on ultrasound monitoring, progesterone can be added, and the embryo can be replaced as described earlier depending on the stage the embryo was cryopreserved. If a pregnancy results, both oestrogen and progesterone are continued until approximately 12 weeks of gestation, beyond which placental hormonal production will maintain the pregnancy.

In the United Kingdom, the current maximum statutory storage period of a cryopreserved embryo is 10 years, but the HFEA permits extension of storage with consent to the gamete provider's 55th birthday if a diagnosis of premature infertility is made.

The rates of pregnancy, miscarriage and congenital anomalies do not appear to be related to the duration of embryo storage. Children conceived from cryopreserved embryos have similar rates of minor and major congenital abnormalities as children conceived naturally.

7.3.7 Success Rates

The HFEA monitors and reports the uptake and outcome of IVF cycles in the United Kingdom. The most recent HFEA report has shown an ongoing increase in both the uptake of and live birth rates with IVF. The report showed that more than a million IVF cycles have now been undertaken in the United Kingdom between 1991 and 2016, with more than 68,000 cycles carried out in 2016.

Female age remains the most important factor in determining the likelihood of fertility treatment outcome. The HFEA data for 2016 showed the national average live birth rate per embryo transfer for women under the age of 35 to be 29% for fresh cycles and 25% for frozen cycles. However, for women of all age groups combined the national average live birth rate per embryo transfer was 21% for fresh cycles and 22% for frozen cycles. The report also showed that the multiple pregnancy rates had come down to 11%, its lowest reported rate in the United Kingdom, without a fall in overall live birth rates.

7.3.8 Risks of IVF

7.3.8.1 Ovarian Hyperstimulation Syndrome
7.3.8.1.1 Clinical Features

OHSS is probably the most serious complication associated with ovarian stimulation. OHSS occurs after the overstimulated ovaries are exposed to hCG, which leads to the production of pro-inflammatory mediators including vascular endothelial growth factor (VEGF). This results in increased vascular permeability within the ovaries, with release of third-space extravascular exudate accumulating within the peritoneal cavity as protein-rich ascites. This shift of fluid into the third space causes a fall in intravascular volume, haemoconcentration and reduced urine output. The expulsion of proteins into the third space exacerbates the drop in intravascular fluid volume.

The severity of ovarian hyperstimulation syndrome can be classified by the degree of fluid accumulation and the extent of biochemical derangement caused. Several schemes have been developed for classifying the severity of OHSS, one such being the Royal College of Obstetricians and Gynaecologists (RCOG) classification. Mild OHSS is characterised by mild abdominal bloating and pain, with ovarian diameter remaining under 8 cm. Moderate OHSS would be considered once ovarian size is measured between 8 and 12 cm, accompanied by ultrasound evidence of ascites as well as symptoms of nausea and vomiting [9].

By the stage the ovaries measure more than 12 cm, there are likely to be features of clinical ascites, oliguria, haemoconcentration as well as biochemical derangement (hyponatraemia, hyperkalaemia, hypoproteinaemia and hypo-osmolality). These findings are consistent with severe OHSS. Critical OHSS occurs when there is continual deterioration in these parameters, leading to tense ascites with large hydrothorax contributing to potential acute respiratory distress and increased risk of thromboembolism. OHSS can potentially be life threatening and deaths have been reported in women with severe or critical OHSS, caused by venous thromboembolism, cerebrovascular thrombosis, renal failure or cardiac tamponade resulting from pericardial effusion.

The incidence of OHSS varies with the different types of fertility treatment. The greater the degree of ovarian stimulation, the greater the risk of OHSS. IVF is thus associated with the highest risk of the complication. The estimated incidence of moderate and severe OHSS combined is approximately 3.1%–8% of all IVF cycles performed. The 14th European IVF-Monitoring report comprising data from 25 European countries found an incidence of hospitalisation rate due to OHSS of 0.3% in 2010.

OHSS can be categorised as either early or late in onset. Early OHSS is typically seen within 7 days of hCG administration, whereas late OHSS occurs beyond 10 days. Late OHSS is usually associated with pregnancy and can be more severe, due to persistent and prolonged stimulation of the ovaries caused by placental hCG production.

Pretreatment risk factors for OHSS include the presence of polycystic ovaries, low body mass index (BMI), younger age as well as previous episodes of OHSS. The appearance of polycystic ovaries in particular is associated with a higher risk of OHSS, perhaps related to differences in accelerated dopamine metabolism in PCOS women compared to normo-ovulatory women. This results in increased vascularisation and higher expression of the signs and symptoms of OHSS.

The use of ovarian reserve markers may also aid the assessment of OHSS risk. A good predictor of OHSS has been elevated serum anti-mullerian hormone (AMH), with levels above 24 pmol/L being particularly at risk. A high antral follicle count (AFC) can also be indicative of risk. The risk of OHSS is estimated to increase from 2.2% in women with an AFC of <24 to 8.6% with an AFC of >24.

7.3.8.1.2 Prevention of OHSS

Ovarian stimulation with low doses of gonadotropins (no higher than 150 IU/day) can reduce the chances of developing OHSS. Meta-analysis data appear to indicate that there is no difference in the risk of OHSS with the various gonadotropins available for ovarian stimulation; however, adopting a short GnRH antagonist protocol for pituitary suppression as opposed to a long agonist has been shown to be associated with a significant reduction in OHSS risk.

The antagonist protocol has a twofold potential benefit in this context. First, lower oestradiol levels are observed during ovarian stimulation, and second it allows for the possibility of triggering ovulation with a GnRH agonist by taking advantage of the flare-up mechanism.

The GnRH agonist induces a rise in serum LH hormone for between 24 and 36 hours, which is adequate for oocyte maturation. This option considerably reduces the incidence of OHSS but is associated with suboptimal luteal development of the endometrium due to the shorter half-life of LH compared to hCG. Studies have shown that live birth rates with a fresh transfer with GnRH agonist trigger appear to be lower than those where hCG trigger has been used. This is likely to be related to inadequate luteal support in the GnRH agonist cycles related to the short half-life of LH. Two approaches have been adopted to overcome this. The first includes elective cryopreservation of all resulting embryos and interval transfer at a later date, referred to as 'the segmentation approach'. The second includes proceeding with a fresh transfer but with additional luteal support either by giving additional oestradiol and progesterone support in the luteal phase or by giving small supplements of hCG in the luteal phase. The latter, though, may result in a small increase in the risk of OHSS. Further research is required to assess the optimal regimen in this context.

The combination of using GnRH antagonist for pituitary suppression and GnRH agonist trigger followed by elective freezing of all resulting embryos with subsequent interval frozen embryo transfer should be considered in women at high risk of OHSS. This is likely to result in a significant reduction in the risk of OHSS without a detrimental effect on live birth outcomes.

Once ovarian stimulation has begun, the presence of more than 20 stimulated follicles signals a high risk of OHSS as well as serum oestradiol levels reaching above 3,500 pg/mL. In these cases, triggering ovulation with an GnRH agonist should be considered. The retrieval of more than 15 oocytes in itself increases the chance of OHSS, and in such cases, elective freezing of all resulting embryos and not proceeding with a fresh transfer should be considered to minimise the risk of late-onset OHSS, the more severe form of the syndrome.

7.3.8.1.3 Management of OHSS

Mild OHSS generally only requires expectant management and maintaining vigilance to detect the possibility of deterioration. A marked increase in weight as well as abdominal distension, nausea and vomiting may signal the onset of moderate OHSS, which requires supportive management in the form of analgesia and fluid management. Severe OHSS generally requires hospital admission, with meticulous fluid balance management, monitoring fluid input and output, measurement of body weight as well as daily monitoring of electrolyte balance, signs of haemoconcentration, liver function test and coagulation profile assessment.

Thromboprophylaxis should be considered to mitigate the increased thrombotic risk and paracentesis may be warranted for symptomatic abdominal ascites. Women with moderate OHSS and selected cases with severe OHSS can be managed on an outpatient management basis including those requiring paracentesis. Women with OHSS being managed on an outpatient basis should, however, have access to urgent review and admission if they develop symptoms or signs of worsening OHSS. In the United Kingdom, fertility treatment centres have an obligation to report adverse incidents including OHSS to the independent regulator, the HFEA.

7.3.8.2 Multiple Pregnancy

The number of multiple births has risen significantly over the past two decades largely due to fertility treatment, as discussed earlier in this chapter. Twin and higher order multiple pregnancies are associated with a higher risk of complications for the mother and baby, and as a result over the last decade the drive in the United Kingdom and many places in Europe and around the world has been to reduce the multiple pregnancy rates largely through a move towards a single-embryo transfer policy.

Twins are six times more likely to be born prematurely, four times more likely to die during pregnancy, five times more likely to die shortly after birth and have a four-fold increased risk of cerebral palsy in comparison with singletons. Moreover, the mother has an increased risk of late miscarriage, high blood pressure, pre-eclampsia, and ante-partum/post-partum haemorrhage.

7.3.8.3 Ectopic Pregnancy

Despite the embryos being transferred into the uterine cavity, patients undergoing IVF still have a risk of an ectopic pregnancy, which may result from the embryo migrating post transfer into the fallopian tubes. This risk is estimated to be between 2% and 5% of IVF cycles.

7.3.8.4 Adverse Obstetric and Perinatal Outcomes

Several studies have assessed obstetric and perinatal outcomes following IVF and ICSI treatment and have reported an increased risk of adverse outcomes. Studies have also shown that infertility itself is associated with an increased risk of adverse obstetric and perinatal outcomes, regardless of whether the couple have had ART treatment.

Pregnant women with a history of infertility, after adjusting for age and parity, have been reported to have an increased risk of pre-eclampsia, placental abruption and placenta praevia and are more likely to require induction of labour, instrumental delivery and Caesarean section compared to controls.

Similarly, singleton pregnancies conceived with IVF, and after controlling for maternal age and parity, have been found to be more likely to develop gestational diabetes, gestational hypertension and placenta praevia. Induction of labour and Caesarean section rates have also been found to be higher.

Perinatal morbidity and mortality appear to be greater in IVF conceived pregnancies with an increased risk of preterm delivery, risk of very low birth weight, small for gestational age babies as well as a higher admission rate to neonatal intensive care.

7.3.8.5 Risks to IVF/ICSI Conceived Children

It is now estimated that more than 5 million babies have been born worldwide through IVF treatment and most long-term follow-up studies of children conceived through IVF and ICSI have so far been reassuring. Many studies have shown no significant differences in psychomotor, cognitive, intellectual or psychological development noted between IVF, ICSI and spontaneously conceived children.

However, large observational studies have reported that babies born after IVF treatment and from spontaneous conception in infertile couples have an increased rate of congenital anomalies of approximately 1%–2% compared to those reported in controls as recorded by the EUROCAT (European Surveillance of Congenital Anomalies network). Anomaly rates with IVF-conceived babies were similar to those conceived spontaneously to infertile couples, suggesting that being infertile is the likely contributory factor to this increase.

7.4 Alternative Assisted Reproduction Treatments

7.4.1 Gamete Intrafallopian Transfer

Gamete intrafallopian transfer (GIFT) involves retrieving oocytes laparoscopically and replacing a number of them into the fallopian tube together with a preparation of highly motile sperm, thus offering the possible advantage of not having the oocytes outside the body for long periods of time.

GIFT was first performed in 1984 and reached peak numbers of procedures performed in the early 1990s. However, GIFT mandated an invasive laparoscopy to replace the oocytes and prepared sperm through the fimbrial end of the fallopian tube. It also offered less information regarding fertilisation and as IVF techniques and success rates improved, the use of GIFT gradually declined.

7.4.2 Zygote Intrafallopian Transfer

Zygote intrafallopian transfer (ZIFT) was introduced in the late 1980s in an attempt to circumvent concerns of poor fertilisation with GIFT. Once the oocytes were retrieved either laparoscopically or transvaginally, they were fertilised in vitro and then transferred back into the fallopian tube.

Similar to GIFT, its role was limited by the need to carry out an invasive procedure and its lower success rates compared to IVF.

7.4.3 Egg Donation

Egg donation involves obtaining oocytes from a healthy donor through controlled ovarian stimulation and fertilising them with the recipient partner's sperm. The resulting embryo(s) will then be transferred back into the recipient's uterus and any surplus good quality embryos can be cryopreserved to use in a future frozen embryo transfer. The recipient's endometrium needs to be synchronised with the donor's ovarian stimulation cycle. This is usually achieved by giving the recipient a combination of oestrogen as well as progesterone to prepare her endometrium for the transfer. Success rates with oocyte donation cycles relate to the age of the donor. The age of the recipient, on the other hand has little impact on the chances of success. The indications for considering egg donation include ovarian insufficiency, either premature or physiological, poor ovarian reserve resulting in repeated IVF failures or in cases where the female partner has a hereditary genetic disease and wishes to avoid genetic transfer to any resulting children. The latter, however, can often be overcome through preimplantation genetic diagnosis.

In the United Kingdom, an egg donor should ideally be less than 36 years old, screened for hepatitis B, hepatitis C and HIV, as well as relevant genetic diseases. Both the recipient and donor should be offered counselling relevant to the implications of egg donation and possible outcomes.

The regulations around donor anonymity in the United Kingdom were changed in April 2005. As a result, children born using donated gametes will be entitled to obtain identifying information about their donor when they reach the age of 18, including the donor's full names, date of birth, their place of birth and their last known postal address. Removal of anonymity has resulted from the recognition that knowledge of the donor's identity is of importance to the donor offspring's psychological development and wellbeing, as has been demonstrated in many studies.

Donors, on the other hand, are entitled to know if any children were born as a result of their donation, the number of children, their sex and year of birth.

There has been a long-standing shortage of egg donors in the United Kingdom that predates the change in anonymity regulations. The change in law with regards to anonymity resulted in an initial decline in the number of egg donors, although these figures have steadily increased over the last decade, suggesting that the removal of anonymity has not negatively impacted people's willingness to donate. This has been in keeping with reported experiences from other countries such as Sweden, where donor anonymity was removed in 1985.

Many patients resort to travelling abroad to have egg donation treatment given the scarcity of donor availability in the United Kingdom, with many having treatment in countries where local regulations maintain donor anonymity.

The HFEA Code of Practice indicates that fertility centres may compensate egg donors with a fixed nominal sum of up to £750 per egg donation cycle to cover their expenses. However, it is not legal in the United Kingdom to pay donors above that, the objective of the latter being to avoid potential exploitation of donors.

Third-party reproduction is discussed in more detail in Chapter 11.

7.4.4 Surrogacy

Surrogacy is an option for women without a functional uterus, either as a result of congenital absence (e.g. Rokitansky syndrome) or after hysterectomy. There are also some women for whom carrying a pregnancy would pose significant medical risk who would benefit from surrogacy.

The woman who delivers the child (the surrogate) remains the child's legal mother until the patient and her partner (the commissioning couple) obtain a formal court order to become the legal parents after the surrogate has delivered. Both the commissioning couple and the surrogate should be counselled as to the implications of treatment, possible outcomes and the legal implications of the process.

The surrogacy process involves obtaining the male partner's sperm and freezing it under quarantine for 6 months, to reduce the transmission risk of hepatitis and HIV infection to the surrogate. A standard IVF

regimen is used, and the surrogate host's endometrium is prepared to receive the resulting embryo in a fashion similar to that with egg donation.

7.5 The Role of the HFEA

The Human Fertilisation and Embryology Authority (HFEA) of the United Kingdom was formed in 1991, following the Human Fertilisation and Embryology Act of 1990. The HFEA grants licences to fertility clinics and monitors practice pertaining to treatment using human gametes and embryos as well as their storage. The HFEA's principal task is to regulate through a system of licensing, audit and inspection, any treatment or research which involves the use and storage of sperm, eggs and embryos for human application. The HFEA also publishes reports on fertility treatment outcomes both for individual clinics as well as reporting national average success rates. This information is available in the public domain. To achieve these standards, fertility centres should have a structure in place that allows them to monitor their processes and outcomes. This should include a clinical governance process and a risk management system as well as having a quality management structure. These measures would allow the centre to monitor the applicability and reproducibility of their pathways as well as their treatment outcomes. It would also allow fertility centres to maintain a set level of standards and improve their service performance.

This is discussed in more detail in Chapter 14.

7.6 Welfare of the Child

The HFEA Code of Practice states that before assisted conception treatment is initiated, an assessment should take place to identify any potential issues that may affect the welfare of any children that may be born as a result of the treatment. Factors that may have an impact on the welfare of a child could be medical or physical risks as well as psychological or social considerations.

7.7 Stopping Treatment

More than half of all IVF cycles started do not result in a successful outcome, and as a consequence, a significant proportion of women and men undergoing fertility treatment do not achieve their desired outcome from treatment. This can be a challenging time and fertility centres have an obligation to ensure that adequate processes are in place to provide patients with information to help guide them through their options and subsequent steps.

Follow-up should be arranged following unsuccessful treatment. The objective of this would be to explain the details of the treatment cycle, offer support and discuss management options and prognosis moving forward. It should also address any queries the couple have.

Going through such a process can be overwhelming for many patients and some may find it difficult to raise all their queries and concerns. It is essential therefore that a sympathetic and facilitative discussion is enabled to cover all issues of relevance, clinical or otherwise.

References

1. NICE guideline: Fertility problems: assessment and treatment. Clinical guideline [CG156]. February 2013.

2. Bhattacharya S, Harrild K, Mollison J, Wordsworth S, Tay C, Harrold A, et al. Clomifene citrate or unstimulated intrauterine insemination compared with expectant management for unexplained infertility: pragmatic randomised controlled trial. *BMJ*. 2008;**337**: a716.

3. HFEA publication on fertility treatment 2014–2016: Trends and figures.

4. Farquhar CM, Liu E, Armstrong S, Arroll N, Lensen S, Brown J. Intrauterine insemination with ovarian stimulation versus expectant management for unexplained infertility (TUI): a pragmatic, open-label, randomised, controlled, two-centre trial. *Lancet*. 2018;**391**(10119):441–50.

5. Al-Inany HG, Youssef MA, Ayeleke RO, Brown J, Lam WS, Broekmans FJ. Gonadotrophin-releasing hormone antagonists for assisted reproductive technology. *Cochrane Database Syst. Rev.* 2016; 4: CD001750.

6. Lensen SF, Wilkinson J, Leijdekkers JA, La Marca A, Mol BWJ, Marjoribanks J, Individualised gonadotropin dose selection using markers of ovarian reserve for women undergoing in vitro fertilisation plus intracytoplasmic sperm injection (IVF/ICSI). *Cochrane Database Syst Rev.* 2018;2:CD012693. DOI: 10.1002/14651858.CD012693.pub2.

7. Chen ZJ, Shi Y, Sun Y, Zhang B, Liang X, Cao Y, et al. Fresh versus frozen embryos for infertility in the Polycystic Ovary Syndrome. *N Engl J Med*. 2016 Aug 11;**375**(6):523–33.

8. Roque M, Haahr T, Geber S, Esteves SC, Humaidan P. Fresh versus elective frozen embryo transfer in IVF/ICSI cycles: a systematic review and meta-analysis of reproductive outcomes. *Hum Reprod Update*. 2019;**25**(1):2–14. DOI: 10.1093/humupd/dmy033.

9. RCOG. Green-top Guideline No. 5: The Management of Ovarian Hyperstimulation Syndrome. February 2016.

Adjuvants in Assisted Reproduction

Chapter

8

Sarah Armstrong and Cynthia Farquhar

8.1 Improving Outcomes in Assisted Reproduction

8.1.1 Introduction

Couples undergoing infertility treatment are a vulnerable population, who are often desperate to optimise any chance of having a baby regardless of the personal and financial cost. For couples undergoing in vitro fertilization (IVF), a plethora of medical and non-medical adjuncts is available; these are known as 'add-ons'. The Human Fertilisation and Embryology Authority (HFEA) defines them as 'optional extras you may be offered on top of your normal fertility treatment, often at an additional cost. They are sometimes emerging techniques that may have shown some promising results in initial studies, or they may have been around for a number of years, but haven't necessarily been proven to improve pregnancy or birth rates.'

ART is a fast-paced area of medicine, with growing demand for treatment, accompanied by rapid innovation which is often driven by industry and pharmaceutical companies. Novel add-on therapies arrive on the market purporting to improve the chance of pregnancy and live birth and they have become established as part of normal working practice in many private clinics, 70% of which offer at least one add-on. Unfortunately, most add-ons are unsupported by good quality randomized evidence. The cost of add-ons is usually borne by patients and provides revenue to the clinics.

Clinics vary with regard to how much information they give patients about whether add-ons have been shown to improve their chance of achieving a much wanted baby, and whether they are cost-effective.

8.1.2 IVF

IVF has been the most advanced and successful treatment option for many infertile couples for almost 40 years. But the success rate from one cycle remains relatively static at approximately 25%–30% (Figure 8.1). This low rate may be an unpleasant surprise for patients.

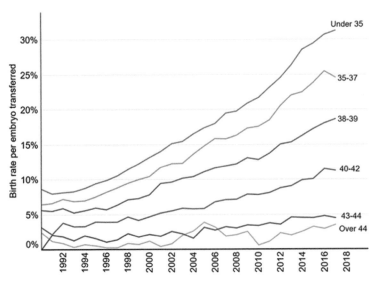

Figure 8.1 Chances of live birth per embryo transferred using patient eggs by age band, 1991–2018.

Reproduced with permission from the HFEA (www.hfea.gov.uk/about-us/publications/research-and-data/fertility-treatment-2018-trends-and-figures/#birthrates)

8.1.2.1 Common Reasons for IVF Failure

A poor response to ovarian stimulation means that women have too few oocytes to collect and use in an IVF cycle. Recurrent implantation failure (RIF) is another common reason for IVF failure: embryos are transferred but pregnancy does not progress. Implantation is one of the most critical steps in determining IVF outcome. It is poorly understood but appears to involve complex signalling and synchronisation between the endometrium and embryo.

Treatment Costs

- NHS funding for IVF varies by region across the United Kingdom, ranging from three funded cycles to none at all.
- IVF is expensive, costing between £3,000 and £5,000 per cycle.
- Approximately 59% of couples self-fund their IVF cycle.
- Most add-ons come at additional cost. This varies enormously between clinics but can be many hundreds of pounds.

8.1.3 The Stance of Professional and Regulatory Bodies on Add-Ons

A British Fertility Society review of the evidence for routine use of IVF adjuncts found that in most cases there was no adequate evidence-based rationale for their use. The sole exception among the interventions that they considered was use of metformin for women with polycystic ovary syndrome undergoing IVF.

The HFEA has created a webpage with consumer-friendly information about the most commonly offered add-ons, with a traffic-light rating system indicating the latest evidence on the efficacy of the most commonly offered add-ons. Red indicates there is no evidence to show that it is effective and safe, amber that there is a small or conflicting body of evidence, meaning further research is still required and the technique cannot be recommended for routine use, and finally, green which indicates that there is more than one good quality randomised controlled trial (RCT) which shows that the procedure is effective and safe.

Currently none of the add-ons assessed by the HFEA are rated green. This means that the HFEA do not think that any of these techniques should be used routinely.

In January 2019 the HFEA and 10 leading professional and patient fertility groups published a consensus statement on add-ons. The key points were as follows: Clinics should offer add-ons only where more than one high-quality study demonstrates a treatment to be safe and effective; clinics should stop offering the treatment add-on if concerns are raised about safety or effectiveness; where evidence is limited or conflicting, clinics offering add-ons should be open with their data to add to the evidence base; where there is no robust evidence, treatment add-ons should be offered only to patients in a research setting; patients must be clearly informed of the experimental nature of any treatment add-on which is offered where there is no robust evidence of its safety or effectiveness; patients should not be charged to take part in a clinical trial; transparent declaration of financial or other interests is essential in discussion with patients.

8.2 Specific Adjuvants

All information on adjuvants discussed in this chapter is based on the latest systematic review and RCT evidence available following database searching (Table 8.1).

Commonly Used Add-Ons

- Surgical
  - Endometrial scratching
- Laboratory
  - Time-lapse imaging of embryos
- Gamete, endometrial and embryological
  - Granulocyte-macrophage colony-stimulating factor (GM-CSF)–containing culture media
  - Assisted hatching
  - Preimplantation genetic testing (PGT-A)
  - Endometrial receptivity array
  - Embryo glue
  - Egg activation with calcium ionophore
  - Intracytoplasmic morphologically selected sperm injection (IMSI)
  - Physiological intracytoplasmic sperm injection (PICSI)
  - Sperm DNA testing
- Medical
  - Reproductive immunology procedures such as
    - Intravenous (IV) immunoglobulin
    - IV lymphocyte immunotherapy
    - IV intralipids
    - Intrauterine granulocyte colony-stimulating factor (GCSF)

Table 8.1 HFEA traffic light coding for add-ons, 2019. Information obtained from https://www.hfea.gov.uk/treatments/treatment-add-ons/

Category	Add-on	Traffic light scoring
Surgical procedures	Endometrial scratching	Amber
Drug therapies	Reproductive immunology	Red
Gamete, endometrial and embryological	Granulocyte-macrophage colony-stimulating factor (GM-CSF)–containing culture media	Amber
	Egg activation with calcium ionophore	Amber
	Assisted hatching	Red
	Embryo glue	Amber
	Preimplantation genetic testing (PGT-A) (on subset of chromosomes)	Red
	Endometrial receptivity array	Amber
	Sperm DNA testing	Amber
	Intracytoplasmic morphological sperm injection (IMSI)	Red
	Physiological intracytoplasmic sperm injection (PICSI)	Red
Laboratory equipment	Time-lapse imaging of embryos	Amber

Key

Green Evidence of clinical effectiveness and safety

Amber Conflicting clinical effectiveness

Red Evidence of clinical ineffectiveness

- Intrauterine peripheral blood mononuclear cells (PBMCs)
- Subcutaneous tumour necrosis factor (TNF)-alpha blocking agents (e.g. adalimumab, infliximab)
- Subcutaneous leukaemia inhibitory factor (LIF)
- Oral steroids (e.g. prednisolone)

8.2.1 Endometrial Scratching

8.2.1.1 Background

Endometrial scratching (or injury), is intentional damage to the endometrium. It is a simple, low-cost outpatient procedure (Figure 8.2) which is sometimes performed prior to IVF or ICSI, particularly in cases of recurrent implantation failure (RIF). It usually involves passing an endometrial pipelle (small sterile flexible plastic tube) through the external os (opening) of the cervix into the uterus.

Potential Advantages

It is hypothesised that endometrial scratching may improve endometrial receptivity, thus making it more likely to lead to embryo implantation. The main proposed mechanisms are:

- Stimulation of decidualisation, a process whereby the endometrium prepares to receive an embryo by modifying stromal cells, uterine glands, uterine vessels and immune cells in order to enhance implantation.
- Stimulation of an inflammatory response with the release of various cytokines and growth factors, which can improve vascularisation and may facilitate embryo implantation.
- Retardation of endometrial maturation, leading to better synchronicity between the embryo and the endometrium. The process of ovarian stimulation for IVF and ICSI leads to abnormal maturation of the endometrium, such that it may be overly mature at the time of embryo transfer and thus less receptive to the embryo.

Potential Disadvantages

- Discomfort, with possible uterine cramping and some bleeding
- Risk of uterine perforation with the pipelle device, and the possibility of infection of the endometrium (endometritis)
- Chance of disturbing a very early spontaneous pregnancy, if endometrial scratching is undertaken in the latter half of a natural menstrual cycle
- Cost (approximately £150)

8.2.1.2 Best Evidence on Clinical Outcomes

In 2019, the largest RCT to date on endometrial scratching for women undergoing IVF was published [1]. More than 1,300 women were randomised to receive an endometrial scratch or no intervention. The primary outcome was live birth. There was no significant difference between the groups in rates of live birth, ongoing pregnancy, clinical pregnancy, multiple pregnancy, ectopic pregnancy or miscarriage. The strengths of this trial include its large sample size, robust allocation concealment and its pragmatic approach across 13 fertility clinics internationally, which improves generalizability of results.

In 2020, the results of the multicentre, RCT 'Endometrial Scratch Trial' were published. 1048 women undergoing their first IVF/ICSI treatment were recruited and randomised to an endometrial scratch in the mid-luteal phase prior to treatment, or to no scratch prior to treatment. Women were aged <37 and expected to be good responders. The findings revealed no difference in livebirth or clinical pregnancy rates between the two arms of the study (livebirth 195/525 in the control arm and 201/523 in the intervention arm, relative risk (RR) 1.03 95% confidence interval (CI) 0.89 to 1.21). The study concluded that endometrial scratch should be ceased in women undergoing their first cycle of IVF/ICSI who are expected to be good responders (2).

The preliminary results of the SCRaTCH study, a multicentre RCT conducted in the Netherlands were published in 2020. In this study, 936 women with one failed IVF/ICSI cycle were randomised to a scratch in the mid-luteal phase prior to ovarian stimulation, or no intervention. The livebirth rate was 22.6% in the scratch group and 18.6% in the control group (RR 1.21, 95% CI 0.94-1.56) (3).

In 2015 a Cochrane review of endometrial scratching was published. It included 14 RCTs (2128 women). The review concluded that endometrial injury performed between day 7 of the previous cycle and day 7 of the embryo transfer (ET) cycle was associated with an improvement in live birth and clinical pregnancy rates in women with more than two previous embryo transfers. There was no evidence of an effect on miscarriage, multiple pregnancy or bleeding and endometrial injury on the day of oocyte retrieval was associated with a reduction of clinical and ongoing pregnancy rates (4).

This review is due to be updated soon, and will include data from the three new large RCTs mentioned above, which may alter its conclusions.

8.2.2 Time-Lapse Imaging

8.2.2.1 Background

Embryos develop in incubation, moving through the fertilisation stage to cleavage stage and on to blastocyst stage in some cases. Embryologists check the developing embryos to select those most likely to implant and develop into a baby. Traditionally, every day the embryo is removed briefly from the controlled environment of the incubator and placed under a light microscope to undergo a morphological check by the embryologist. Time-lapse imaging allows the embryologist to monitor the developing embryo without removing it from the incubator and to select the best embryo for transfer based on the timing and synchronicity of early mitotic divisions and abnormal cleavage patterns that generate morphokinetic parameters. There has been widespread uptake of TLS in IVF clinics worldwide.

Potential Advantages

- The availability of detailed digital images of developing embryos, which can be compiled to create a time-lapse sequence of their development
- Achievement of an undisturbed culture environment for embryos, which avoids exposing embryos to mechanical disturbance or changes in temperature, pH, humidity and gas composition
- The availability of embryo selection software, with complex algorithms based on a combination of

morphokinetic parameters and selection and de-selection criteria which help the embryologist to select the optimal embryo for transfer

Potential Disadvantages

- Exposure of embryos to light during the acquisition of digital images of embryos, often as frequently as every 5–10 minutes. Although the total dose of ultraviolet radiation is likely to be very low, there is potential for harm, which could influence clinical outcomes such as miscarriage and stillbirth. However, overall light exposure is thought to be lower than with traditional embryo assessment under a light microscope.
- Costs approximately £850

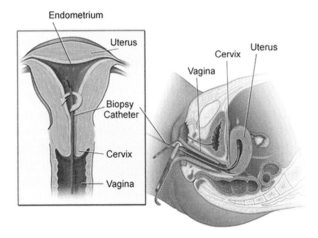

Figure 8.2 The endometrial biopsy procedure.
Image provided by Krames Staywell, 780 Township Line Road, Yardley, PA 19067.

8.2.2.2 Best Evidence on Clinical Outcomes

A 2019 Cochrane systematic review included nine RCTs (2,955 women) and concluded that there was insufficient good quality evidence of differences in live birth or ongoing pregnancy, miscarriage, stillbirth or clinical pregnancy to choose between TLS, with or without embryo selection software, and conventional incubation [4]. The evidence was low or very low quality overall because of a high risk of bias in two studies secondary to lack of adequate randomisation and allocation concealment, indirectness because of the largest study using donor oocytes from young women and imprecision of the results, with broad confidence intervals stretching from significant benefit to significant harm.

8.2.3 Assisted Hatching

8.2.3.1 Background

Assisted hatching involves thinning the zona pellucida (the coat surrounding the fertilised egg), or making a hole in it, using acid or lasers.

> **Potential Advantages**
> - It is suggested that failure of the zona pellucida to rupture following blastocyst expansion may be a contributing factor in failure of embryo implantation and that thinning the zona pellucida may assist the embryo to 'hatch'.

> **Potential Disadvantages**
> - Assisted hatching may increase the risk of multiple pregnancy and there is also a potential risk of damage to the embryo.

8.2.3.2 Best Evidence on Clinical Outcomes

A 2012 Cochrane review of 31 RCTs demonstrated that while assisted hatching does appear to offer a significantly increased chance of achieving a clinical pregnancy (the level only just reached statistical significance: odds ration [OR] 1.13; 95% confidence interval [CI] 1.01–1.27, moderate quality evidence), the 'take-home' baby rate was not proven to be increased [2]. This is mainly due to most trials failing to report on live birth rates. When restricting analysis of clinical pregnancy rate to those trials that went on to report live birth, which on the whole were better quality trials with a lower risk of bias, the clinical pregnancy result showed insufficient evidence of a difference between the assisted hatching and the control group.

Overall, there was some evidence of increased multiple pregnancy in the assisted hatching group. The quality of the evidence is overall poor to moderate secondary to selective reporting in a number of studies and significant statistical heterogeneity between trials.

The National Institute for Health and Care Excellence (NICE) recommends against the use of assisted hatching because of lack of evidence of benefit.

8.2.4 Preimplantation Genetic testing

8.2.4.1 Background

Preimplantation genetic testing for aneuploidy (PGT-A) entails chromosomal analysis of embryos and transfer only of those diagnosed as euploid (normal). Various assessment techniques have been used, including fluorescence in situ hybridization (FISH), comparative genomic hybridization (CGH), array CGH (aCGH), digital polymerase chain reaction (dPCR), single-nucleotide polymorphism (SNP) array, real-time quantitative PCR (qPCR) and next-generation sequencing (NGS). Older types of PGT-A assessed only a limited subset of chromosomes, whereas current techniques assess all 23 pairs of chromosomes. Costs and timing vary, but few of these technologies allow for fresh embryo transfer.

Potential Advantages

- PGT-A identifies aneuploid embryos that are unsuitable for fertility treatment (as they are unlikely to develop into a baby or may result in a baby being born with a genetic condition).

Potential Disadvantages

- Possible false-positive results, leading to loss of healthy embryos
- Possible false-negative results, leading to an abnormality being missed
- Possible embryo damage, causing developmental problems in the womb or in later life
- High cost

8.2.4.2 Best Evidence on Clinical Outcomes

A 2011 Cochrane review included nine RCTs of PGT-A. All used FISH technology to assess a subset of chromosomes, a method that is now rarely used. The review found that PGT-A significantly *decreased* live birth rates in women with a poor prognosis and was not associated with a benefit in any population [4].

A 2018 evidence review by the American Society for Reproductive Medicine (ASRM) found three relatively small RCTs conducted in couples with a favourable prognosis, one RCT conducted in women of advanced age and several retrospective cohort studies. Although some studies reported higher birth rates after aneuploidy testing the ASRM concluded that the value of PGT as a universal screening test for all IVF patients has yet to be determined. The Cochrane review is in the process of being updated and will include evidence from the latest RCTs on the topic.

8.2.5 Endometrial Receptivity Array

8.2.5.1 Background

The endometrial receptivity array (ERA) involves testing of an endometrial biopsy sample to establish whether the endometrium is receptive to embryo transfer. It is proposed as an investigative test for selected women with repeated implantation failure (RIF). It purports to identify women whose 'window of opportunity' for embryo transfer is 'altered' (i.e. does not fall within days 19–21 of the menstrual cycle).

Potential Advantages

- Improvement of implantation rates in women with RIF with good quality embryos and a normal uterus and endometrium

Potential Disadvantages

- Delay of embryo transfer until the following cycle
- Invasive nature of test, which might disrupt implantation
- Cost

8.2.5.2 Best Evidence on Clinical Outcomes

A 2018 RCT reported that a policy of personalised embryo transfer using the ERA resulted in an increased implantation rate in Japanese women with RIF, compared with deferred embryo transfer ($n = 506$) [5].

An interim analysis of an industry-sponsored RCT ($n = 356$) revealed that there was no difference in pregnancy rate per embryo transfer between fresh or deferred embryo transfer in women undergoing their first IVF/ICSI cycle. In addition, this study appears to never have published its completed results [6]. Currently there is no randomised evidence to show that ERA is associated with significantly increased rates of ongoing pregnancy or live birth.

8.2.6 GM-CSF–Containing Culture Media

8.2.6.1 Background

GM-CSF is a cytokine (growth factor) produced by epithelial cells in the uterus and fallopian tubes, with receptors on human embryos and the ovary. It appears to exert a positive control over various genetic paths and may have survival-promoting effects on embryos.

Potential Advantages

- GM-CSF supplementation of culture media may improve IVF success rates by promoting embryo development and increasing implantation rates.

Potential Disadvantages

- The promotion of rapid cell proliferation by GM-CSF could theoretically be associated with loss of

  genomic imprinting, which could increase the risk of genetic and/or chromosomal abnormalities in the offspring.
- Culture medium with growth factor is more expensive than standard media and may cost an additional £420–£440.

8.2.6.2 Best Evidence on Clinical Outcomes

A systematic review of CM-CSF–containing media included four RCTs and concluded that there was no clear evidence that they improve pregnancy and live birth rates [7]. No meta-analysis was performed and only one study reported live birth rates. Study quality was not explored and it is unclear how many women were randomised in each study. A subsequent RCT also found no clear evidence of benefit [8]. A Cochrane review on GM-CSF containing culture media was published in 2020. It included five studies, three of which were able to be meta-analysed (1532 participants). The review concluded that there was very low to low quality evidence of uncertainty whether GM-CSF containing culture media was any more or less effective than culture media not supplemented with GM-CSF for clinical outcomes that reflect effectiveness and safety. Furthermore, the claims from marketing information that GM-CSF has a positive effect on pregnancy rates are not supported by the available evidence in the review [4].

8.2.7 Embryo Glue (Hyaluronic Acid)

8.2.7.1 Background

Hyaluronic acid (HA) is used as a supplement to conventional embryo transfer medium, with the aim of improving implantation rates via the following proposed mechanisms: HA may indirectly promote angiogenesis and improve of cell-to-cell and cell-to matrix adhesion, thus assisting in embryo apposition and attachment to the endometrium; the high viscosity of HA may enhance embryo transfer and prevent expulsion of embryos from the uterine cavity after transfer; and HA may act as a receptor mediation, as the primary HA receptor is CD44, which is also expressed in the preimplantation embryo and in the endometrium.

Potential Advantages

- The rate of human implantation is innately low (10%–30%) and failed implantation is a common

  cause of IVF failure. Any improvement in the implantation rate may maximise the chance that infertile couples can achieve pregnancy and livebirth. Improved implantation rates may also lead to a reduction in the need to replace multiple embryos in IVF and reduce the risk of multiple pregnancy.

Potential Disadvantages

- A raised multiple pregnancy rate is the expected natural consequence of increased implantation and pregnancy rates. This suggests that clinics using HA-supplemented embryo transfer medium should re-evaluate their elective single-embryo transfer policy, closely monitor their multiple pregnancy rate and ensure that patients are aware, not only of the possible increased chance of pregnancy, but also of the increased chance of multiple pregnancy if multiple embryos are transferred.

8.2.7.2 Best Evidence on Clinical Outcomes

A 2015 Cochrane review included 16 RCTs ($n = 3,687$) using transfer medium supplemented with HA and reported moderate quality evidence of improved clinical pregnancy and live birth rates. However, multiple pregnancy rates were also increased, possibly due to a combination of adherence compound with a policy of multiple embryo transfer in most studies [4]. Only six studies reported live birth rates; however, the meta-analysis is dominated by one large RCT of good quality. Evidence was overall of moderate quality, with evidence of statistical heterogeneity between studies and most studies being deemed at high risk of bias in at least one aspect.

A subsequent RCT compared HA versus conventional transfer medium in 581 cycles and found no evidence of a benefit in pregnancy or live birth rates [9].

8.2.8 Artificial Egg Activation with Calcium Ionophore

8.2.8.1 Background

Egg (oocyte) activation is a cascade of intracellular processes triggered by the fertilising spermatozoa which initiates the transition from oocyte to embryonic development and prevents fertilisation by multiple sperm. Activation failure can be associated with sperm or oocyte deficiencies such as poor ovarian response, nonmotile spermatozoa or poor sperm morphology, but can also occur with good quality sperm and oocytes. Oocyte activation failure may account for 40%–70% of unfertilised oocytes exposed to ICSI. Oocyte activation can be stimulated artificially, most commonly by chemicals called calcium ionophores which can be added to the embryo in the lab.

Potential Advantages

- Calcium ionophores can potentially induce oocyte activation and thus increase the chance of a successful pregnancy for couples with a history of total fertilisation failure or low fertilisation.

Potential Disadvantages

- There are ethical concerns about the use of artificial egg activation because this intervention bypasses natural regulatory measures and could theoretically cause epigenetic defects during the preimplantation incubation period. Patients undergoing this treatment need to be carefully selected and the rationale for treatment needs to be well justified. Oocyte or sperm donation may present a reasonable treatment alternative for some couples.

8.2.8.2 Best Evidence on Clinical Outcomes

A systematic review of AOA found no properly randomised RCTs that utilised calcium ionophores

in couples with fertilisation failure [10]. There are also no follow-up studies on the safety of this technique.

8.2.9 Intracytoplasmic Morphologically Selected Sperm Injection (IMSI)

8.2.9.1 Background

Sperm micromanipulation, such as intracytoplasmic morphologically selected sperm injection (IMSI), is used for treatment of male infertility associated with reduced sperm concentration or motility. In ICSI, one sperm is selected under high magnification (×200–600) and injected directly into the oocyte. A newer method of sperm selection selects the sperm under ultra-high-powered (×6,000) magnification.

Potential Advantages

- Ultra-high-powered magnification allows detection of some organelle malformations that are not otherwise evident. It is suggested that

  intracytoplasmic morphologically selected sperm injection (IMSI), using spermatozoa selected under high magnification, may increase pregnancy rates in couples with repeated implantation failures.

Potential Disadvantages

- There are no specific safety issues associated with the use of IMSI in addition to ICSI.

8.2.9.2 Best Evidence on Clinical Outcomes

A Cochrane review of nine RCTs (2,014 couples) compared regular ICSI with IMSI [4]. There was no evidence that use of IMSI influenced live birth or miscarriage, though there was very low quality evidence to suggest a benefit in pregnancy rates. Only one small study reported live birth, with very serious imprecision of the estimate. The quality of the evidence for miscarriage and clinical pregnancy was very low owing to high risk of bias related to differing embryo transfer numbers between the groups, imprecision in the estimate and inconsistency across the included studies. In addition, a strong indication of publication bias was suspected.

8.2.10 PICSI

8.2.10.1 Background

Physiological intracytoplasmic sperm injection (PICSI) is a technique that aims to improve the selection of the best sperm for injection into the egg. In PICSI, sperm are selected based on their ability to bind HA, which occurs naturally in the cumulus–oophorus complex. Such sperm may have better indicators of genomic integrity, including lower levels of deoxyribonucleic acid fragmentation, chromosomal aneuploidy and cytoplasmic retention and hence increased maturity.

> **Potential Advantages**
>
> - PICSI might potentially facilitate selection of the best quality sperm, thus reducing the likelihood of miscarriage and increasing the live birth rate in couples undergoing ICSI.
> - HA selection could potentially be beneficial to couples for whom semen quality is too poor for IVF and may also have a significant benefit for older women with poorer quality eggs that have a decreased potential to repair sperm DNA damage.
>
> **Potential Disadvantages**
>
> - There are no specific safety issues associated with the use of PICSI (as opposed to conventional ICSI).

8.2.10.2 Best Evidence on Clinical Outcomes

A Cochrane review found only one RCT (n = 482) comparing PICSI versus conventional ICSI and found no clear benefit from use of PICSI [4]. A subsequent RCT of 156 couples with unexplained infertility and normal semen parameters also found no evidence of benefit from PICSI [11]. A recent RCT compared PICSI versus ICSI in 2,722 couples undergoing an ICSI procedure and found that PICSI offered no clear advantage in relation to the primary outcome. PICSI led to a reduced miscarriage risk, but had no effect on pregnancy rates or preterm live birth rate [12].

8.2.11 Sperm DNA Test

8.2.11.1 Background

Conventional semen analysis does not assess all aspects of the function of testis and sperm quality. Sperm DNA fragmentation tests are proposed as a new means of testing the functional competence of the sperm, by measuring the level of DNA damage in sperm. Sperm DNA can potentially 'be'? damaged during sperm development and storage in the epididymis, or as a result of endogenous metabolic by-products or exogenous toxins such as cigarettes.

> **Potential Advantages**
>
> - New tests for predicting the likelihood of pregnancy after IVF or ICSI would be clinically useful as part of fertility work-up.
>
> **Potential Disadvantages**
>
> - Sperm DNA tests are performed using a semen sample. They are thus non-invasive and do not incur significant additional risk to the patient.

8.2.11.2 Best Evidence on Clinical Outcomes

A systematic review included 30 diagnostic studies evaluating the value of sperm DNA tests for predicting ongoing pregnancy with IVF or ICSI [13]. Tests included were the sperm chromatin structure assay (SCSA), sperm chromatin dispersion (SCD) test, terminal deoxynucleotidyl transferase mediated deoxyuridine triphosphate nick end labelling (TUNEL) and single electrophoresis (Comet) assay. The SCSA and the SCD test have a poor predictive value, and the TUNEL assay and Comet assay have a fair predictive value. The tests had little or no difference in predictive value between IVF and ICSI.

Routine use of sperm DNA fragmentation tests cannot be recommended in couples undergoing IVF or ICSI, either for the prediction of pregnancy or for the choice of treatment. The evidence was limited by heterogeneity between the studies and serious methodological weaknesses, and the authors recommend further research.

8.2.12 Reproductive Immunology Procedures

8.2.12.1 Background

Immunological disorders have been suggested as a cause of adverse IVF outcomes, especially when no other cause can be identified. Various immunomodulators have been used, including intravenous (IV) immunoglobulin, IV lymphocyte immunotherapy, IV intralipids, intrauterine granulocyte colony-stimulating factor (GCSF), intrauterine peripheral blood mononuclear cells (PBMCs), subcutaneous TNF-alpha blocking agents (e.g. adalimumab, infliximab), subcutaneous leukaemia inhibitory factor (LIF) and oral steroids (e.g. prednisolone).

Potential Advantages

- It is suggested that immunomodulators may improve IVF success rates by improving uterine receptivity, enhancing implantation and preventing early miscarriages.

Potential Disadvantages

Reproductive immunology treatments suppress the body's natural immunity and have various risks. For example:

- Immunoglobulin: headache, muscle pain, fever, chills, low back pain and rarely thrombosis (blood clots), kidney failure, anaphylaxis
- Intralipids: headache, dizziness, flushing, nausea, possible clotting or infection
- TNF-alpha blocking agents: infections including septicaemia, chronic infections such as tuberculosis and severe allergic reactions to the

drug. Remicade (infliximab) is not recommended for use during pregnancy.
- Steroids: high blood pressure, diabetes and premature birth

8.2.12.2 Best Evidence on Clinical Outcomes

A Cochrane systematic review of 14 RCTs (n = 1,879) using peri-implantation corticosteroids in IVF or ICSI cycles found no evidence of an increase in live birth rates, though there was some evidence of increased pregnancies in women having IVF [4].

A 2013 systematic review reported higher pregnancy and live birth rates from using intravenous immunoglobulin in women with repeated implantation failure, but this review included case-control studies [14].

A 2018 systematic review included 15 RCTs ($n = 1,855$) of women undergoing IVF or ICSI and considered the evidence on all commonly used immunomodulators. There was no evidence that immunomodulators improve live birth rates in women undergoing IVF treatment, with or without a history of RIF, and no long- or short-term safety data were available. The authors

suggested that immunotherapy should be used only in the setting of a clinical trial [15].

8.3 Conclusion

Reproductive medicine is a fast paced and emotive area of medicine, where innovation is often driven by patient demand and financial considerations. It is recognised that novel interventions and technologies often enter fertility clinics without appropriate development and evidence to demonstrate their safety and efficacy. In most cases the add-ons described in this review entered the clinical setting prior to large multisite RCTs, and certainly before clinical and cost-effectiveness was established.

All too often patients are paying for add-ons to ART cycles that are potentially ineffective or even harmful, and which can be very expensive. Such adjuncts must be investigated with properly powered, well-designed RCTs, which can then be incorporated into systematic reviews. If (as seems all too likely) novel technologies continue to be adopted into clinical practice prior to adequate investigation, it is beholden upon clinicians to seek out the latest randomised evidence and ensure that patients are well informed and aware of the uncertainly regarding such treatments. This is necessary to guide decision-making in both patients and clinicians, in the face of strong industry marketing.

References

1. Lensen S, Osavlyuk D, Armstrong S, Stadelmann C, Hennes A, Napier E, et al. A randomized trial of endometrial scratching before in vitro fertilization. *N Engl J Med*. 2019;**380**(4):325–34.

2. Metwally MC, R; Pye, C; Dimairo, M; White, D; Walters, S; Cohen, J; Chater, T; Pemberton, K; Young, T; Lomas, E; Taylor, E; Laird, L; Mohiyiddeen, L; Cheong, Y. Endometrial scratching in women undergoing their first In Vitro Fertilisation (IVF) cycle: results from the UK Multicentre Endometrial Scratch Randomised Controlled Trial. ESHRE: Human Reproduction; 2020. p. i140.

3. Van Hoogenhuijze, N. Torrance, H.L.; Eijkemans, M.J.C.; Broekmans, F.J.M. (2020). Twelve-month follow-up results of a randomized controlled trial studying endometrial scratching in women with one failed IVF/ICSI cycle (the SCRaTCH trial). ESHRE: Human Reproduction; 2020.

4. Cochrane. Cochrane Library 2019. Available at: www.cochranelibrary.com

5. Taguchi S, Funabiki M, Hayashi T, Tada Y, Iwaki Y, Karita M, et al. The implantation rate of Japanese infertile patients with repeated implantation failure can be improved by endometrial receptivity array (era) test: a randomized controlled trial. *Fertil Steril.* 2018;**110**(4):e90.

6. Simon C, Vladimirov IK, Castillon Cortes G, Ortega I, Cabanillas S, Vidal C, et al. Prospective, randomized study of the endometrial receptivity analysis (ERA) test in the infertility work-up to guide personalized embryo transfer versus fresh transfer or deferred embryo transfer. *Fertil Steril.* 2016;**106**(3):e46-e7.

7. Siristatidis C, Vogiatzi P, Salamalekis G, Creatsa M, Vrachnis N, Glujovsky D, et al. Granulocyte macrophage colony stimulating factor supplementation in culture media for subfertile women undergoing assisted reproduction technologies: a systematic review. *Int J Endocrinol.* 2013;**2013**:704967.

8. Sfontouris IA, Anagnostara K., Kolibianakis EM, Lainas TG. Effect of granulocyte-macrophage colony-stimulating factor (GM-CSF) on pregnancy rates in patients with multiple unsuccessful IVF attempts. *Hum. Reprod.* 28(Suppl 1):i60–i62.

9. Fancsovits P, Lehner A, Murber A, Kaszas Z, Rigo J, Urbancsek J. Effect of hyaluronan-enriched embryo transfer medium on IVF outcome: a prospective randomized clinical trial. *Arch Gynecol Obstet.* 2015;**291**(5):1173–9.

10. Sfontouris IA, Nastri CO, Lima ML, Tahmasbpourmarzouni E, Raine-Fenning N, Martins WP. Artificial oocyte activation to improve reproductive outcomes in women with previous fertilization failure: a systematic review and meta-analysis of RCTs. *Hum Reprod.* 2015;**30**(8):1831–41.

11. Majumdar G, Majumdar A. A prospective randomized study to evaluate the effect of hyaluronic acid sperm selection on the intracytoplasmic sperm injection outcome of patients with unexplained infertility having normal semen parameters. *J Assist Reprod Genet.* 2013;**30**(11):1471–5.

12. Kirkman-Brown J, Pavitt S, Khalaf Y, Lewis S, Hooper R, Bhattacharya S, et al. Sperm selection for assisted reproduction by prior hyaluronan binding: the HABSelect RCT. Efficacy and Mechanism Evaluation. Southampton, UK: NIHR Journals Library, 2019.

13. Cissen M, Wely MV, Scholten I, Mansell S, Bruin JP, Mol BW, et al. Measuring sperm DNA fragmentation and clinical outcomes of medically assisted reproduction: a systematic review and meta-analysis. *PLoS ONE.* 2016;**11**(11):e0165125.

14. Li J, Chen Y, Liu C, Hu Y, Li L. Intravenous immunoglobulin treatment for repeated IVF/ICSI failure and unexplained infertility: a systematic review and a meta-analysis. *Am J Reprod Immunol.* 2013;**70**(6):434–47.

15. Achilli C, Duran-Retamal M, Saab W, Serhal P, Seshadri S. The role of immunotherapy in in vitro fertilization and recurrent pregnancy loss: a systematic review and meta-analysis. *Fertil Steril.* 2018;**110**(6):1089–100.

Laboratory Procedures for Assisted Reproduction

Virginia N. Bolton

9.1 Background

From the time of ovulation and fertilisation until the developing embryo reaches the uterus and implants some days later, the mammalian embryo is a free-floating entity within the female genital tract. It is this unique feature that has made the development of assisted reproduction therapies possible. The earliest studies, undertaken in the rabbit and mouse, led developmental biologists to develop culture conditions that allowed the successful fertilisation of eggs in vitro (literally 'in glass'), the culture of developing embryos and finally embryo transfer, culminating in the first live birth following IVF and embryo transfer, in the mouse, in 1958.

The transposition of skills and techniques developed in the animal research laboratory to clinical application in the treatment of infertility has entailed decades of refinement of the early techniques for achieving successful fertilisation and embryo culture in vitro. The introduction of legislation and associated regulations in the United Kingdom (the Human Fertilisation & Embryology Act 1990; amended in 2008) and Europe (the EU Tissues and Cells Directive), guidelines from professional bodies [1, 2] and the drive to improve success rates have led to the development of relatively sophisticated laboratories and procedures that serve this sector today.

9.2 The Laboratory Environment

The impact of variables such as patient demographics, ovarian stimulation regimens and clinical oocyte recovery on gamete quality are outside the control of the laboratory practitioners. However, once the patient's gametes have been passed to the laboratory, the primary objective is to maintain constant and consistent conditions, within prescribed acceptable ranges, in order to minimise any damage that may compromise their viability. A consistent, optimised environment in the laboratory, within individual workstations and critical items of equipment; the consistent performance of individual practitioners; and the selection of appropriate culture media, reagents, equipment and consumables will all have a critical bearing on treatment outcomes (Table 9.1).

Minimising variation in every element within the assisted reproduction laboratory is ensured through the implementation of a quality management system (QMS [3]). Hazards that must be controlled include exposure to infectious organisms and environmental toxins, to fluctuations in temperature and pH and to physical damage sustained during manipulation and micromanipulation.

Monitoring and regulation of environmental variables are achieved using an accurate, objective monitoring system with associated alarms, ensuring that critical equipment functions within prescribed ranges at all times. This includes the monitoring of temperature in all working areas (heated stages in laminar flow hoods; microscope stages), incubators, fridges and freezers and tanks of liquid nitrogen (Dewars) in which cryopreserved material is stored. In addition, mechanisms should be in place to monitor the levels of individual gases within incubators.

9.2.1 The Cryostore

The hazards associated with the use of liquid nitrogen mean that as well as compulsory safety training and equipment to protect staff, the tanks of liquid nitrogen (Dewars) used for storing cryopreserved embryos and gametes must be located separately from, but in close proximity to the assisted reproduction laboratories. Oxygen monitors, and associated audible and visible alarms, must be installed in the cryostore to alert staff both inside and outside the laboratory suite to potentially fatal low atmospheric oxygen. Appropriate flooring material, that can withstand cryodamage caused by spillages of liquid nitrogen, must be installed.

Table 9.1 Factors affecting outcome in the assisted reproduction laboratory

Building/construction	Non-toxic materials, glues, paints
	Filtered lighting to block UV irradiation
Design	Proximity to clinical areas
	Ergonomically designed to maximise efficiency and minimise risk
	Restricted access for designated staff
	Storage for consumables
	Disposal of waste
	Adjacent cryostore
Air quality (minimum Grade D; optimally Grade C or higher [1])	Positive pressure
	HEPA filtered
	Activated carbon filters to reduce volatile organic carbons (VOCs)
Critical equipment	Laminar flow hoods (vertical laminar flow; Class II)
	Refrigerators
	Incubators
	Warmed worksurfaces/test tube holders
Culture media	Core components:	Water
		Salts (maintain osmolality)
		Energy substrate
		Buffer (pH 7.2–7.4)
		Protein supplement
	Gas phase and buffers in air:	HEPES or MOPS buffer
		In incubators: sodium bicarbonate buffer and 5%–6% CO_2
		Low O_2 (5%) in incubators is recommended
Staff competency	Training and assessment
	Adherence to standard operating procedures (SOPs)
	Attention to detail

9.2.2 Witnessing

To prevent any mismatches of gametes or embryos, it must be possible to identify unambiguously every sample of gametes or embryos at all stages of the laboratory and treatment processes. Meticulous systems must be in place, so that each step involving the movement of gametes or embryos between containers (test tubes, petri dishes and cryopreservation holding devices) is witnessed. To minimise the risk of involuntary automaticity during witnessing, it is recommended that an objective, electronic witnessing system, such as bar coding or radio frequency identification (RFID), should be used for every step where it is physically possible.

9.3 Use of Sterile Working Areas Within the Laboratory

Laminar flow hoods must be used in the laboratory wherever a sterile working area is required. The type of hood used for different workstations in the

laboratory depends upon the level of protection against microbial contamination required (Figure 9.1).

Class II cabinets provide protection for the operator and the environment as well as for the product. These hoods must be used for procedures when the operator is handling body fluids (follicular fluid, blood, semen) including

- Oocyte retrieval
- Surgical sperm collection
- Semen analysis
- Semen preparation
- Semen cryopreservation and warming
- Thawing cryopreserved semen/surgically collected sperm

Vertical or horizontal laminar flow hoods provide protection for the product and equipment, but not for the operator or the environment. These hoods are used for all procedures where containers (petri dishes/flasks/vials/test tubes) of culture medium and reagents that contain, or will be used to contain

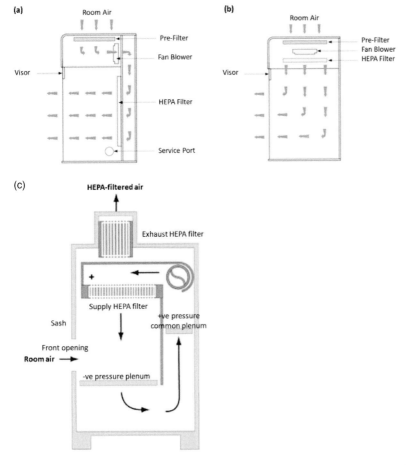

Figure 9.1 Diagrams illustrating air flow in vertical or horizontal laminar flow and Class II hoods. *Laminar flow* hoods provide protection for the product but not the operator. (a) Horizontal laminar flow. (b) Vertical laminar flow. Room air is drawn into the high-efficiency particulate air (HEPA) filter; 99.99% particle-free air is forced across the work surface. (c) *Class II* hoods provide protection for the product, the operator and the environment.

gametes and/or embryos are open to the atmosphere, including

- Preparation of culture tubes and dishes
- Decanting media and reagents
- IVF insemination
- All procedures when oocytes/embryos are moved between dishes
- Denudation of oocytes
- Intracytoplasmic sperm injection (ICSI)
- Embryo biopsy
- Cryopreservation of oocytes and embryos
- Thawing/warming of oocytes and embryos

9.4 Use of Buffers in Culture Media

Dishes and test tubes of culture medium for use in gamete preparation and embryo culture are prepared using sterile techniques in laminar flow hoods and must be warmed to 37°C before use. Medium in culture dishes may be overlaid with pharmaceutical grade light mineral oil, to minimise temperature, osmolality and pH fluctuations in the medium, especially when dishes are exposed to the atmosphere during procedures outside the incubator.

9.4.1 Working in Air

When carrying out procedures outside the incubator, such as during oocyte retrieval and ICSI, if the procedure entails working at the microscope for any length of time, it is common to use media that are buffered with HEPES or MOPS, which maintain physiological pH in atmospheric levels of CO_2.

9.4.2 Culture in Incubators

Incubators are maintained with an atmosphere of 5%–6% CO_2 and culture media used for incubation are buffered with sodium bicarbonate. With bicarbonate-buffered culture medium, CO_2 dissolves into the medium and reacts with water to form carbonic acid according to the Henderson–Hasselbalch equation (Figure 9.2). The concentration of sodium bicarbonate in the culture medium must be matched with the level of CO_2 in the atmosphere in the incubator to achieve the appropriate, physiological pH.

Dishes and tubes of bicarbonate-buffered medium must be allowed to equilibrate in the incubator before use, usually overnight but at least for several hours, depending on the volumes of medium used, in an

$$HA(aq) \rightleftharpoons A^-(aq) + H^+(aq)$$

Weak acid   Conjugate base

$$pH = pKa + \log \frac{[A^-]}{[HA]}$$

[HA] concentration of the weak acid
[A]   concentration of its conjugate base
pKa of the weak acid

Figure 9.2 The Henderson–Hasselbalch equation: pH of buffers.

atmosphere of between 5% and 6% CO_2 according to the concentration of sodium bicarbonate in the medium.

9.5 Oocyte Retrieval

Oocyte retrieval must be carried out in a Class II laminar flow hood, which provides protection not only to the environment and the product, but also for the operator working with body fluids. Aspirated follicular fluid is collected into test tubes held in a warmed, monitored heated block maintained at 37°C. Tubes of follicular fluid are passed from the operating theatre to the (ideally) adjacent laboratory, where the bloodstained fluid is tipped into a shallow petri dish on a surface warmed to 37°C and examined for the presence of oocyte–cumulus complexes (OCCs) (Figure 9.3).

Working at a stereomicroscope with a warmed stage within the Class II laminar flow hood, using sterile technique, each OCC is aspirated gently using a polished Pasteur pipette and rinsed through petri dishes containing fresh, warmed culture medium before being placed into labelled dishes. Each dish is witnessed and uniquely identified as that of the patient undergoing the procedure. Dishes containing OCCS are placed into an incubator positioned adjacent to the workstation.

The pH of the culture medium used, of which numerous products are commercially available, is maintained using the appropriate buffer to maintain physiological pH in the working environment (Table 9.1).

Appropriate decontamination procedures must be carried out between each patient's oocyte retrieval procedure.

9.6 Semen Analysis and Sperm Preparation for Insemination In Vitro

The sperm for insemination may be prepared from fresh or frozen (cryopreserved) semen, or from fresh

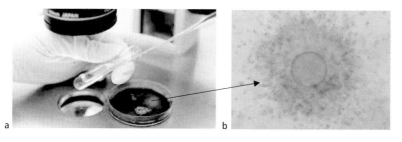

a   b

Figure 9.3 Oocyte retrieval: visualisation of the oocyte–cumulus complex. (a) Oocyte retrieval: using a sterile Pasteur pipette, the follicular fluid is expelled into a petri dish on the warm stage of a stereomicroscope in a Class II laminar flow hood; the oocyte–cumulus complex can be seen with the naked eye in the blood-stained fluid. (b) The oocyte within the oocyte cumulus complex, as visualised using the stereomicroscope.

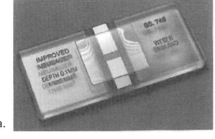
a.

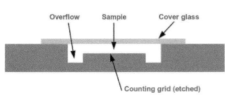
b.

c.

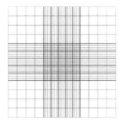

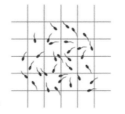
d.

Figure 9.4 Use of the Neubauer counting chamber for sperm concentration assessment. (a) The Neubauer counting chamber. Note the Newton's rings between the coverslip and the chamber; the appearance of the Newton's rings confirms that the coverslip is attached appropriately, the chamber depth is fixed correctly, and the sperm concentration assessment will be accurate. (b) Diagrammatic representation of the side view of the counting chamber. (c) Diagrammatic representation of the counting grid of the chamber as visualised using the microscope. (d) Diagrammatic representation of a higher magnification of the counting grid with sperm suspension ready for concentration assessment.

or frozen (cryopreserved) surgically collected sperm samples. Samples must be processed in a Class II laminar flow hood, as for oocyte retrieval, to provide protection for the operator as well as for the environment and the sample [4].

9.6.1 Semen Analysis

Before preparation, samples are assessed for sperm concentration, motility and morphology [5]. Routine semen analysis should be carried out using phase contrast microscopy, and motility analysis using warmed microscope stages at 37°C. Ideally, bright field microscopy should be available for the examination of sperm morphology. Neubauer haemocytometers should be used for assessing sperm concentration (Figure 9.4). Alternative counting chambers are available (e.g. Makler) but are less accurate.

Computer-assisted semen analysis (CASA) may be used to reduce inter-operator variation, but where this is not available, the subjective nature of most aspects of semen assessment mean that it is important to carry out internal quality assurance for all semen analysis practitioners within each laboratory, in conjunction with regular external quality assurance exercises, such as the UK National External Quality Assessment Service (NEQAS), both to assess performance and to minimise variation between and within laboratories.

9.6.2 Sperm Preparation

Sperm must be prepared before use in insemination in vitro, to remove the seminal fluid, non-sperm cells and contaminating micro-organisms from fresh and cryopreserved semen samples. Preparation will yield a concentrated suspension of sperm, in culture medium, with improved motility, and may enhance the concentration of those with normal morphology.

All procedures are carried out using sterile technique in a Class II laminar flow hood, and care is taken throughout preparation to protect sperm samples from extreme fluctuations in temperature and pH. Appropriate decontamination procedures must be carried out between processing samples from different patients. To avoid the risk of cross-contamination and mismatches between patients, laboratory staff should process one sample at a time, and at each step during preparation where the sample is transferred between containers, unique identifying labels on each matching container must be witnessed.

Sperm is most commonly prepared using either a buoyant density gradient centrifugation or 'swim-up' technique (Figure 9.5), although for severely oligozoospermic or cryptozoospermic samples (Table 9.2) where few motile sperm are present, other techniques may be used.

9.6.2.1 Buoyant Density (Isopycnic) Centrifugation

This separation technique relies on the different buoyant densities of cells and debris in the sperm sample (semen; surgically collected testicular sperm; post-ejaculatory urine in cases of retrograde ejaculation). Separation according to buoyant density is achieved by centrifugation of the sample for 20 minutes at 300 g (1,500–1,600 rpm) on a discontinuous,

Table 9.2 WHO reference values for normal semen [5]

Parameter	WHO criteria	Diagnosis if criteria not met	
Volume	≥1.5 mL	*Aspermia* (where there is no ejaculate); possible *retrograde ejaculation*	
Appearance	Grey and opaque		
pH	≥7.2		
Concentration (× 10^6/mL)	≥15	*Oligozoospermia*	*Cryptozoospermia* (sperm only seen after centrifugation); *azoospermia* (no sperm present)
Motility (% progressive)	≥32	*Asthenozoospermia*	*Necrozoospermia* (only dead sperm present)
Normal morphology (%)	≥4	*Teratozoospermia*	*Globozoospermia* (round heads; no acrosome)
Leucocytes (× 10^6/mL)	≤1	Infection	

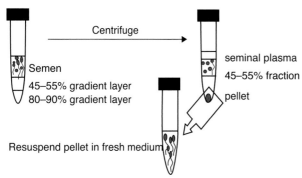

Figure 9.5 Sperm preparation: buoyant density centrifugation.

two-layer gradient of colloidal silane-coated silica particles (usually 80%–90% and 45–55% suspensions in HEPES- or MOPS-buffered medium). Motile, morphologically normal spermatozoa become concentrated at the bottom of the gradient, and can be collected for use in insemination, leaving immotile, abnormal forms, cells and other contaminants elsewhere in the column.

9.6.2.2 Swim-Up

Up to 1 mL of warmed, equilibrated bicarbonate-buffered culture medium is carefully layered over the semen sample in a test tube. Alternatively, the semen sample may be first diluted 1:2 with warmed, equilibrated medium, and the suspension centrifuged for 10 minutes at 1,500 rpm. After discarding the supernatant, the pellet (20–50 μL) is gently resuspended and overlaid with 1 mL of fresh warmed, equilibrated culture medium. With both approaches, the test tube of sperm overlaid with culture medium is placed, inclined at an angle of 45°, in an incubator at 37°C in an atmosphere of 5% or 6% CO_2 as appropriate for the culture medium used. After incubation for approximately 1 hour, the upper layer of culture medium is collected and transferred into a fresh tube.

9.6.2.3 Wash and Spin

In cases of severe oligozoospermia (<0.1 × 10^6/mL) and cryptozoospermia (Table 9.2) it may be appropriate simply to centrifuge the entire sample, diluted at least 1:2 with warmed, equilibrated culture medium, in order to concentrate the small number of sperm present into a 20- to 50-μL pellet.

9.6.3 Sperm Vitality Tests

Where sperm are present in the sample, but few or no motile forms are seen, it is possible to assess whether or not any of the immotile forms are viable using sperm vitality tests. Such tests determine the proportion of live, membrane-intact spermatozoa, either by dye exclusion (e.g. eosin–nigrosin staining) or by osmoregulatory capacity demonstrated by swelling of the sperm tail under hypo-osmotic conditions (the hypo-osmotic swelling [HOS] test). Sperm staining techniques destroy living cells and can only be used diagnostically, but the HOS test does not affect sperm viability and may be used on samples intended for use in treatment.

9.6.4 Chemical Motility Enhancers

Where so few or no motile sperm are seen after preparation of a sample, such that there will be difficulty finding sufficient motile forms to carry out ICSI, the motility of immotile, viable spermatozoa may be stimulated using preparations containing a chemical motility enhancer (pentoxifylline or theophylline). These members of the xanthine family inhibit phosphodiesterase activity and increase levels of intracellular cyclic adenosine monophosphate (cAMP), which plays a role in sperm motility. Clinical grade preparations of chemical motility enhancers are available commercially, specifically for use in assisted reproduction procedures. Their addition to immotile sperm in samples such as surgically retrieved epididymal or testicular sperm samples may induce motility, significantly reducing the time taken to identify and select motile sperm for use in ICSI. Fertilisation, pregnancy and live birth can be achieved with treated sperm, but use of chemical motility enhancers should be restricted to cases where it is considered essential by the experienced ICSI practitioner; where live births have been reported following pentoxifylline or theophylline treatment, there is no evidence of anomalies in the offspring, but larger follow-up studies are needed to confirm their safety.

9.7 Insemination In Vitro

9.7.1 Conventional Insemination (IVF)

For normal semen samples [5] (Table 9.2), it is usual practice to inseminate OCCs at approximately 4–6 hours after oocyte retrieval using conventional IVF. Usually, up to five OCCs will be incubated in 1 mL of culture medium. With gametes for only one set of patients in a workstation at any time, and with appropriate witnessing, insemination is carried out at a stereomicroscope with a warmed stage at 37°C in a laminar flow hood, using a graduated pipette with a sterile, disposable tip that must be discarded between patients. An appropriate volume of the prepared, concentrated sperm suspension (usually 5–20 µL) is expelled into each drop of culture medium containing OCCs, to give an insemination concentration of $50–100 \times 10^3$/mL motile spermatozoa. The mixed OCCs and spermatozoa are incubated overnight, and the oocytes checked for evidence of fertilisation 18–20 hours post insemination.

9.7.2 Intracytoplasmic Sperm Injection

First described in 1992, ICSI is now an established technique used routinely in the assisted reproduction laboratory. ICSI involves the selection and injection of a single motile spermatozoon into each mature oocyte in a cohort in order to maximise the chance of fertilisation where

- Initial semen analysis shows the sample is suboptimal in one or more parameters (Table 9.2).

- Sperm have been collected surgically (epididymal or testicular) [6].
- Frozen semen samples have shown poor survival on thawing.
- The final sperm preparation intended for use in IVF insemination does not meet the laboratory's criteria for conventional IVF.
- A clinically significant titre of antisperm antibodies is present.
- Previous IVF treatment cycle(s) have resulted unexpectedly in complete fertilisation failure.
- Cryopreserved oocytes are used.

No definitive guidelines have been developed for the routine use of ICSI to achieve fertilisation in vitro outside these criteria. Although its efficacy when used for other indications remains disputed, ICSI may be used routinely in some assisted reproduction centres for

- Unexplained infertility
- Women of advanced maternal age (usually ≥40 years)
- Where oocyte quality is deemed to be poor according to the laboratory's own criteria
- Patients whose embryos showed poor development in previous treatment cycle(s)

9.7.2.1 Preparation of Oocytes for ICSI

Prior to ICSI, the cumulus and corona radiata cells surrounding each oocyte must be removed in a procedure known as denudation, usually carried out 3–4 hours after oocyte retrieval. Using sterile technique and appropriate witnessing, working in a laminar flow hood at a stereomicroscope with a warmed stage at 37°C, the first stage of denudation is enzymatic digestion of the matrix of hyaluronan oligosaccharide chains cross-linked by hyaluronan binding proteins and proteoglycans between the cumulus granulosa cells and oocyte. The OCCs are incubated in hyaluronidase for 30–45 seconds, after which any remaining cumulus and corona radiata cells are removed mechanically, using fine (0.01 mm internal diameter) pipettes. Clinical grade human recombinant hyaluronidase is available commercially, specifically for use in oocyte denudation for assisted reproduction, and is usually added to HEPES- or MOPS-buffered culture medium, since dishes containing oocytes may be exposed to air for several minutes during the procedure.

Once denuded, each oocyte can be assessed for maturity using a stereomicroscope, and those that are mature (metaphase II stage of meiosis; MII), as indicated by the extrusion of the first polar body, are selected for injection (Figure 9.5). Oocytes that are still at the germinal vesicle (GV) stage will usually degenerate in culture without undergoing maturation in vitro and are discarded. Any MI oocytes may be returned to culture in the incubator and examined at intervals throughout the day of oocyte retrieval. Those that mature to the MII stage, extruding the first polar body after further incubation, may be added to the patient's cohort to be used for ICSI. MII and MI oocytes are returned to fresh dishes of warmed, pre-equilibrated bicarbonate-buffered medium before they are returned to the incubator for incubation until ICSI is performed, at around 4–6 hours following oocyte retrieval.

9.7.2.2 Preparation of the Micromanipulation Workstation

For ICSI it is necessary to use an inverted phase microscope with higher magnification than the stereomicroscope (up to ×40 objectives), fitted with a warmed stage at 37°C, and Hoffman modulation contrast optics to enhance the image. The ICSI rig (Figure 9.6) should be housed within a laminar flow hood to maintain sterility. Micromanipulators intrinsic to the rig, adjusted using coarse and fine control joysticks, are connected to micro-syringes that regulate aspiration and expulsion through fine, polished glass pipettes: a blunt, relatively large holding pipette (external diameter~80–120 µm; internal diameter~17–35 µm), usually on the left, and a smaller sharpened and bevelled injection needle (external diameter ~6–7 µm; internal diameter ~4.5–5.5 µm), usually on the right. The two micropipettes must be inserted into the holders carefully and securely to establish the necessary seal, and they must be aligned in the correct horizontal plane with precision, both individually and in apposition to each other, to ensure ease of injection and minimise damage to the oocyte. Once their correct insertion and alignment has been confirmed, levers attached to the holders are used to elevate the micropipettes before placing the ICSI dish onto the warm stage of the microscope, maintained at 37°C. Each set of micropipettes must be removed and discarded after each ICSI procedure.

9.7.2.3 Preparation of the ICSI dishes

For ICSI, shallow petri dishes are used, and prepared using sterile technique in a laminar flow hood with droplets (5–10 µL) of culture medium, usually HEPES- or MOPS-buffered for procedures carried out in air. If bicarbonate-buffered medium is used, prepared ICSI dishes must be pre-equilibrated in the incubator in an atmosphere of 5%–6% CO_2 as appropriate before use. Working on a cool surface to reduce evaporation, droplets of culture medium are expelled onto the centre of the base of the dish, to form a circle of droplets surrounding a central ~5 µL droplet of polyvinylpyrrolidone (PVP) suspended in culture medium; the viscous PVP suspension causes the motile sperm to move more slowly, facilitating their capture for use in injection, and is also used to 'prime' the microinjection needle, thereby controlling the rate of injection of the spermatozoon into each oocyte to minimise damage through accidental expulsion of large volumes. Droplets are overlaid with mineral oil, and the prepared ICSI dish is warmed to 37°C.

9.7.2.4 The ICSI Procedure

Immediately prior to ICSI, working with appropriate witnessing at a stereomicroscope with a warmed stage at 37°C in a laminar flow hood,~2 µL of prepared sperm suspension is added to the central PVP droplet, and an MII stage oocyte is placed into each of the surrounding droplets of culture medium in the prepared, warmed ICSI dish. The dish is placed on the warm stage of the inverted phase microscope at the ICSI rig, and the micropipettes are lowered from their elevated position into the dish, to rest at the level of the oocytes. In order to prevent gametes sticking to the inside of the micropipettes, and to

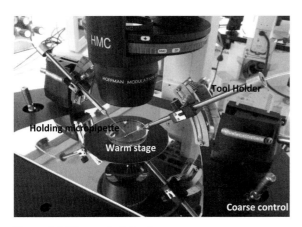

Figure 9.6 Micromanipulation rig.

prevent inadvertent expulsion of air bubbles into the droplets, the holding pipette is 'primed' by aspirating culture medium, and the microinjection pipette is 'primed' by aspirating PVP, using the microsyringes connected to the holders.

Using ×400 magnification to visualise the spermatozoa in the drop of PVP, a motile, morphologically normal sperm is targeted and immobilised by lowering the microinjection pipette over its tail, close to the midpiece, and swiftly 'slashing' the pipette across it, pressing it against the base of the dish. Immobilisation in this way is necessary to reduce damage that may be caused by introducing a motile spermatozoon into the ooplasm of the oocyte, but is also thought to allow the release of sperm cytosolic factors through the ruptured tail membrane, thereby eliciting oocyte activation after injection.

9.7.2.5 ICSI

Once immobilised, the spermatozoon is aspirated, tail first, in a minimum volume of PVP suspension, into the microinjection pipette, and the ICSI dish is moved on the microscope stage so that the first oocyte for injection can be visualised. Injection of the spermatozoon into the oocyte can then proceed (Figure 9.7). After each oocyte in the dish has been injected, the oocytes are moved, with appropriate witnessing, into fresh culture dishes of warmed, pre-equilibrated bicarbonate-buffered medium and incubated overnight.

9.7.2.6 Techniques to Refine the Criteria for Selection of Sperm for Use in ICSI

The criteria for selection of sperm for ICSI, according to motility and morphology assessed using ×400 magnification, are relatively crude and subjective. This raises the concern that any inherent selection mechanisms that function in natural conception, and to an extent in conventional IVF, that may have evolved to ensure that abnormal sperm are de-selected and excluded from fertilising oocytes are overridden by the laboratory practitioner practising ICSI. While it remains possible that this concern may apply in cases of extremely abnormal semen samples, ICSI has been practised widely and routinely worldwide since 1992, and no comparisons of live birth rates and offspring lend significant weight to this concern.

Nonetheless, it remains possible that in certain cases, the inadvertent selection of abnormal sperm for use in ICSI may contribute to the poor development of embryos that fail to implant, or that miscarry after establishing a pregnancy, and therefore techniques are available [7], although not yet used widely, for selection of sperm using more sophisticated criteria (Table 9.3).

9.8 Assessment of Fertilisation

Whether they have been mixed with sperm using IVF or ICSI, oocytes are examined 18–20 hours later for evidence of fertilisation. For oocytes that have been

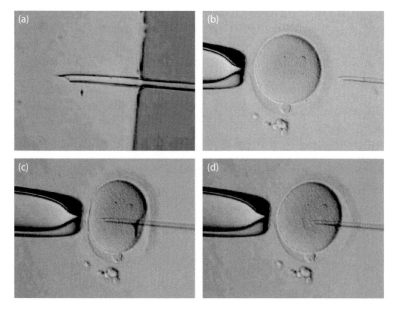

Figure 9.7 ICSI. (a) An immobilised spermatozoon is aspirated from the droplet of PVP into the injection micropipette. (b) The MII oocyte is orientated with the polar body at 6 o'clock or 12 o'clock, held by gentle vacuum applied to the holding pipette; the injection micropipette with the aspirated spermatozoon is aligned at 3 o'clock in the same plane, and the sperm is expelled so it is held at the tip of the injection micropipette. (c) The injection micropipette is pushed through the zona pellucida (the glycoprotein matrix that forms a protective coating for the oocyte) to the centre of the oocyte, ensuring the tip does not reach the oolemma adjacent to the holding pipette; a gentle vacuum is applied with the microsyringe attached to the microinjection pipette, to aspirate the oolemma until it ruptures, at which point the vacuum is immediately released. (d) The spermatozoon is injected into the ooplasm with the minimum volume of PVP and the injection micropipette is withdrawn.

Source: K Coward and D Wells (eds), *Textbook of Clinical Embryology* (Cambridge University Press, 2013).

Table 9.3 Techniques to refine criteria for sperm selection for use in ICSI

Technique	IMSI	PICSI/HABSelect
Meaning	Intracytoplasmic morphologically selected sperm injection	Physiological intracytoplasmic sperm injection Hyaluronic acid binding sperm selection
Rationale	Vacuoles in sperm heads negatively affect embryo quality and outcome	Only mature, structurally sound sperm have capacity to bind to hyaluronan
Selects	Sperm with confirmed normal head organelles	Sperm that demonstrate ability to bind to hyaluronan
Requirement	High-power microscope (×6,600)	Petri dishes coated with hyaluronan
Suggested benefit	Improve rates of live births, clinical pregnancy, implantation, embryo quality, fertilization; reduce miscarriage rate	Improve rates of live births, clinical pregnancy, implantation, embryo quality, fertilization; reduce miscarriage rate
Drawbacks	Very time consuming Technically challenging Expensive equipment; occupies laboratory space No evidence for impact on live birth or miscarriage rates	Moderately time consuming Technically challenging Moderate additional expense of consumables
Quality of Evidence	Limited evidence for improved clinical pregnancy rate Too weak to recommend routine use	Good evidence from large multicentre RCT shows no impact on live birth rate per couple

inseminated with conventional IVF, any remaining cumulus and corona radiata cells not digested away by the hyaluronidase released from the sperm acrosomes must be removed before this is possible. Working in a laminar flow hood, at a stereomicroscope with a warmed stage, residual cells are removed mechanically using a fine pipette.

Denuded oocytes following IVF and ICSI are assessed for the presence of pronuclei, two pronuclei indicating that normal fertilisation has occurred. Using sterile technique and with appropriate witnessing, oocytes with two pronuclei are separated and moved into fresh dishes of warmed, pre-equilibrated culture medium and returned to the incubator.

Oocytes with no pronuclei have either not fertilised because they are still immature (GV or MI stage; Figure 9.8), or pronuclei have failed to develop normally despite penetration of an MII oocyte by the spermatozoon. Oocytes with more than two pronuclei have fertilised abnormally with more than one spermatozoon penetrating the oocyte (polyandry), or have failed to extrude the second polar body after resumption of meiosis II (polygyny) (Figure 9.9). The presence of a single pronucleus may indicate that the oocyte has become activated parthenogenetically.

9.9 The Challenge of Failed Fertilisation

With conventional IVF, even where all semen parameters are within the normal range (Table 9.2), complete

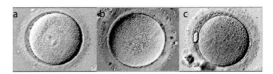

Figure 9.8 Stages of maturation of human oocytes. Denuded human oocytes; diameter 0.01 mm. (a) Germinal vesicle stage. (b) Metaphase I (MI). (c) Metaphase II (MII).

failed fertilisation of all the oocytes in a cohort may result unexpectedly, in around 2%–5% of treatment cycles. Even with ICSI, failed fertilisation may occur in around 2% of cycles. This unanticipated, devastating premature end to a patient's treatment has prompted exploration of mechanisms [7] to ameliorate the impact in the same treatment cycle (rescue ICSI) or to ensure it does not happen in a subsequent treatment cycle (using ICSI after unexplained failed fertilisation with conventional IVF; using artificial oocyte activation after no oocytes develop pronuclei following ICSI).

9.9.1 Rescue ICSI

In cases in which all or most in a cohort of oocytes have failed to fertilise following conventional IVF, 'rescue ICSI' is sometimes performed in countries outside the United Kingdom on the day after oocyte retrieval. This practice is not permitted in the United Kingdom, as its safety is unproven. Safety concerns include those associated with the fertilisation of aged oocytes, whose

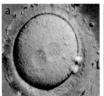
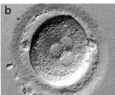
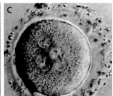

Figure 9.9 Normal and abnormal fertilization. (a) Normal (two pronuclei). (b) Abnormal (three pronuclei). (c) Abnormal (multiple pronuclei).

chromosomes may have become disrupted, and the fact that some oocytes that do not display evidence of fertilisation when assessed after IVF may nonetheless have been penetrated by sperm. In the absence of sufficient data, the theoretical risk of generating abnormal embryos for use in treatment with this practice has been deemed too great by the UK regulator, the Human Fertilisation and Embryology Authority (HFEA), for it to be permitted.

9.9.2 Artificial Oocyte Activation

Calcium ionophores such as A23187, or compounds such as strontium chloride, are used increasingly to activate oocytes artificially in the assisted reproduction laboratory, when fertilisation has failed in an earlier ICSI cycle. Such agents cause a single, transient increase in intracellular calcium, rather than reproducing the physiological calcium oscillations seen with normal oocyte activation at fertilisation. Nonetheless, this non-physiological single calcium peak is sufficient to achieve fertilisation and has been used successfully clinically, in cycles with previous fertilisation failure due to severe male factor infertility, or due to deficient oocyte maturation and/or development. However, until adequate information is available from follow-up studies, in particular with respect to possible epigenetic consequences or effects on gene expression in resulting offspring, artificial oocyte activation must be considered experimental and should be applied only when appropriately indicated.

9.10 Embryo Culture

The fertilised oocytes remain in culture in the incubator to allow the embryos to develop until the time of embryo transfer or cryopreservation. Throughout the culture period, until the embryos have either been transferred to the uterus, cryopreserved and placed into storage for later use, or deemed unsuitable for use in treatment and discarded, it is mandatory that the conditions they are exposed to in vitro mimic as

closely as possible physiological conditions (Table 9.1). This is achieved through the use of carefully selected, maintained and monitored equipment.

9.10.1 Incubators

The critical equipment for embryo culture is the incubator, which must be selected for its ability to maintain the medium for culturing gametes and embryos at 37°C in a constant gas phase to achieve physiological pH in the bicarbonate-buffered culture medium, with fluctuations following frequent opening and closing of the door kept to a minimum. Different categories of incubator may be used, each with properties suited to specific functions in the assisted reproduction laboratory (Table 9.4).

9.10.2 pH

Maintaining physiological pH through the use of appropriate media, buffered according to whether used for carrying out procedures in air, or for culture in an atmosphere of high CO_2 in the incubator, is critical. The developing embryos must be maintained at physiological pH in order to facilitate normal:

- Gene expression
- Metabolic and enzyme activity
- Maintenance of gap junctions
- Maintenance of the cytoskeleton
- Modulation of calcium levels
- Cell proliferation

9.10.3 Gas Phase

Embryo culture in the incubator may be in atmospheric (20%) or reduced (5%) oxygen. High oxygen has been found to have adverse effects on embryo development in several animal species, where the negative impact of oxidative stress on cellular metabolism, gene expression and differentiation is well established. Evidence is accumulating to support the use of low oxygen in the clinical assisted reproduction

Table 9.4 Incubators used in the assisted reproduction laboratory

Incubator type	Relative recovery rate after door opening		Specific properties	Appropriate for:
	Gas phase	Temperature		
Chest (front-loading)	Slow	Slow	Large Spacious Repeated, frequent door opening during long recovery time exposes contents to relatively long periods of suboptimal temperature and pH	Pre-equilibration of media Sperm preparation
Benchtop (top-loading)	Immediate	Fast	Compact Purges with pre-mixed gas restoring steady state gas phase rapidly after door opened/closed Base of culture dish in direct contact with warm surface to maintain/restore steady-state temperature	Culture of oocytes and embryos Dishes removed for assessment of development
Time lapse	Fast	Fast	Compact Allows undisturbed culture	Oocyte and embryo culture; Dishes remain in situ for assessment of development Morphokinetic analysis

setting, but some scepticism remains concerning its benefits, and low oxygen in human embryo culture has yet to be adopted universally.

9.10.4 Culture Media

Many different culture media are available commercially. Their precise constituents and/or their concentrations are not always specified, but all aim to enhance culture conditions by uniquely supplementing the product with essential and non-essential amino acids, vitamins and even growth factors and cytokines. There is no conclusive evidence to support the selection of one of those available over any of the others.

While the core constituents of culture media remain largely unchanged between commercial products, specific changes in practice in the use of different categories of media have been incorporated as laboratory practices have evolved:

- A *universal medium* was used initially for all embryo culture. This was during a time when embryo survival beyond day 3 was poor, with only ~20% of fertilised oocytes surviving in vitro and developing into blastocysts on day 5.

  ○ For this reason, embryo transfer was performed routinely during cleavage stages (day 2/3 after fertilisation in vitro).

- *Sequential media* were introduced during attempts to improve the rate of embryo survival in vitro beyond day 3. The rationale behind use of these media was that

  ○ Stage-specific media provide different metabolic substrates tailored to meet the specific requirements of the embryo at different stages of development (*sodium pyruvate* during fertilisation and cleavage stages up to day 3; *glucose* from day 3 onwards).

  ○ They were initially thought to be essential for successful extended culture of embryos beyond day 3.

  ○ Their use encouraged the introduction into routine clinical practice the culture of embryos until development to the blastocyst stage (day 5).

  ○ The drive to avoid multiple pregnancy while maintaining acceptable overall successful pregnancy rates, through transfer of a single embryo rather than two or even three

embryos, required that the single embryo for transfer can be selected from a cohort with confidence.

  ○ Improved selection of the single 'best' embryo from a cohort for transfer is possible if embryo transfer is delayed until viable embryos develop into blastocysts; non-viable embryos undergo arrest/degeneration in vitro by day 5 or 6.

- *Single-step medium*: The concept of using a single medium for all stages of development has been revisited and introduced recently to

  ○ Maximise the benefit of using incubators incorporating time lapse imaging technology, which allow observation and assessment of embryo development without disturbing culture conditions

  ○ Acknowledge that the improved standard of all aspects of performance of assisted reproduction laboratories is conducive to embryo survival, and that the use of sequential media may have been a 'red herring'

  ○ Provide greater understanding of embryo resilience, whereby the embryo is able to select and utilise specific constituents from the culture medium as and when required, provided they are all present at appropriate concentrations

9.11 Strategies for Embryo Selection and Embryo Transfer

The culmination of all the laboratory procedures in assisted reproduction is the embryo transfer, the goal of which is to maximise the chance of achieving pregnancy and a healthy singleton live birth. Two key factors to consider with respect to embryo transfer are (1) how best to select from within a cohort the most viable embryo(s) for transfer [8], and (2) how many embryos to transfer [9].

9.11.1 Embryo Selection

9.11.1.1 Conventional Assessment

Historically, selection has been according to grading systems that allocate embryos a quality score according to their rate of development and overall morphology, as visualised at the level of the light microscope. This remains the most widely used routine method of evaluation. Morphological assessment of each embryo

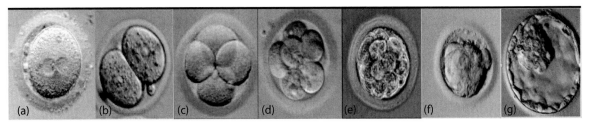

Figure 9.10 Preimplantation stages of the human embryo. (a) Normally fertilised oocyte 18–20 hours post insemination, day 1. (b)–(d) Cleavage stages, days 2–3. (e) Compacting, day 4. (f) Compacted morula, day 4. (g) Expanded blastocyst, day 5.

is made using a stereomicroscope with a warmed stage at a fixed time on day 3, during cleavage and, where embryos are left in culture until those that have the capacity to do so undergo blastocyst formation, again on day 5 (Figure 9.10). The subjectivity of embryo assessment means that it is important to carry out internal quality assurance for all practitioners within each laboratory, ideally in conjunction with regular external quality assurance exercises, such as the UK NEQAS and GameteExpert scheme, to assess individual performance within the laboratory, and to minimise variation within and between laboratories.

During each cleavage division, between days 1 and 3 after oocyte retrieval and fertilisation, the cells (blastomeres) of the embryo halve in size, while the embryo itself remains the same size (0.1 mm diameter). Cleavage stage embryos are scored according to the rate of cell division (two-cell stage by late day 1/early day 2; four-cell stage by day 2; eight-cell stage by day 3), and the symmetry, size and extent of fragmentation of the blastomeres (Figure 9.11a).

Late on day 3, the embryo begins to undergo compaction, where the outlines of individual blastomeres can no longer be distinguished, and the morula stage embryo forms on day 4. Junctions between the embryo's cells form a seal and the cells begin to differentiate; fluid accumulates in the blastocoelic cavity and the blastocyst forms, which is the earliest stage of development where different cell types can be distinguished in the embryo: the inner cell mass (ICM) surrounded by an outer layer of trophectoderm cells. As the blastocoel expands, the blastocyst begins to increase in size, and continues to do so until it hatches from the thinned zona pellucida, the point at which, in vivo, implantation begins.

The number and quality of the cells in these two cell types, the ICM and trophectoderm, and the degree of expansion of the blastocoel, are the criteria by which blastocysts are scored on day 5 (Figure 9.11b).

9.11.1.2 Time Lapse Imaging

A more sophisticated, less subjective evaluation of embryo viability involves morphokinetic analysis, made possible with the introduction of time lapse incubator technology. Time lapse incubators are in use in many assisted reproduction centres, a number of which use algorithms derived in their laboratories using morphokinetic data from time lapse imaging to augment conventional morphological evaluation for embryo selection. Currently there is insufficient evidence that time lapse imaging analysis is superior in embryo selection compared with conventional methods. Well-designed RCTs are needed to evaluate fully the effectiveness of such algorithms in clinical use. It remains possible that the coincidental benefit of uninterrupted culture afforded by time lapse incubators, where there is no need to open the incubator and remove embryos in order to assess their morphology (Table 9.4), may reduce the potential for damage to embryos in vitro, thereby improving embryo survival.

9.11.2 How Many Embryos to Transfer, and When

A strategy for embryo selection and embryo transfer must have sufficient flexibility to take into consideration the differences between individuals and couples undergoing treatment. Each assisted reproduction centre will, through audit of its own experience and evaluation of published data, develop criteria for its embryo transfer strategy that maximise the chance of a healthy singleton live birth for a varied population. These criteria will take into consideration:

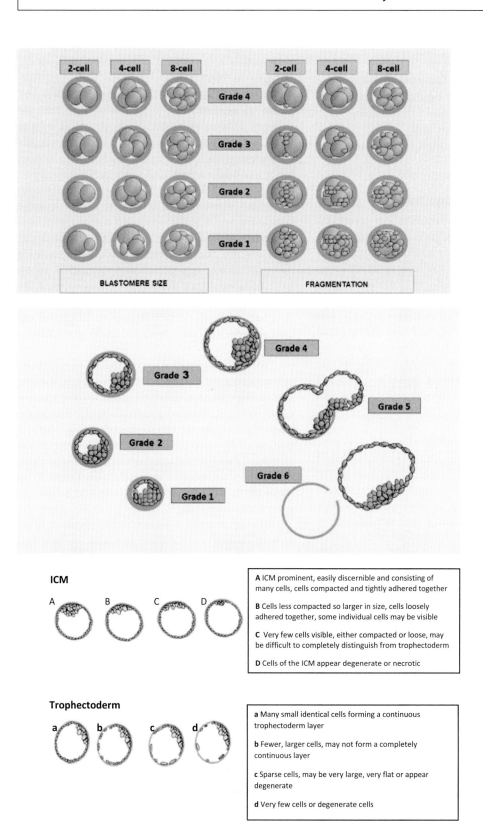

Figure 9.11 Schematic illustrations of embryo morphology and grading [13]. (a) Days 2–3 (cleavage stages). (b) Day 5–6 (blastocyst stage): expansion of the blastocoelic cavity. (c) Day 5–6 (blastocyst stage): quality of the two cell types (inner cell mass [ICM] and trophectoderm).

- The female partner's age
- The indication for treatment
- The number of previous failed treatment cycles
- Whether or not there has been a previous pregnancy, either spontaneous or following assisted reproduction treatment
- The number and quality of the embryos in the present cohort

9.11.2.1 Elective Single-Embryo Transfer

A single embryo may be transferred in treatment cycles where more than one good quality embryo is available, and where there are additional embryos in the cohort that are considered suitable for cryopreservation, for use in a subsequent treatment cycle. Commonly, eSET will be practised in cycles with relatively good prognosis (first treatment cycle; female partner is ≤38 years old) [9]. Embryos are assessed on day 3 after fertilisation, and if there is more than one good quality embryo in the cohort, they will be left in culture until day 5, when a single blastocyst will be selected for transfer and any remaining blastocysts cryopreserved.

9.11.2.2 Double-Embryo Transfer

Up to two embryos may be transferred in cycles in which the prognosis is less good (previous failed treatment cycle(s); female partner ≥39 years old) and/or where there is only ≤1 good quality embryo in the cohort, assessed on day 3 after fertilisation; in such cases it is common to proceed with embryo transfer on day 3, rather than wait until day 5.

9.11.2.3 Triple-Embryo Transfer

This is only permitted in the United Kingdom where the female partner is ≥40 years old and using her own oocytes rather than those donated by a younger woman. Increasingly, however, double-embryo transfer or even eSET is used routinely for this group of women, particularly in their first treatment cycle, to avoid the risk of twin or triplet pregnancy.

9.12 Cryopreservation

Cryopreservation is the preservation of structurally intact living cells and tissues using very low temperatures. Semen cryopreservation has been carried out successfully, and has been part of routine clinical practice, since 1953 and does not merit further consideration here.

The first successful pregnancy following cryopreservation and thawing of a human embryo was reported in 1983, 5 years after the birth of Louise Brown in 1978, and embryo cryopreservation is now routine in assisted reproduction, with frozen-thawed embryos yielding pregnancy rates almost as high as those with fresh embryos. In contrast, successful oocyte cryopreservation has taken longer to master, but it was finally recognised as a reliable clinical procedure in 2012 and is now included among techniques performed routinely in the assisted reproduction laboratory. Successful embryo and oocyte cryopreservation has enabled maximisation of the live birth rate from a single oocyte retrieval procedure, providing the confidence to implement a systematic eSET policy, so that while the 'time to pregnancy' may increase, the multiple birth rate is reduced. Oocyte cryopreservation has led to the establishment of successful egg banking for oocyte donation and for fertility preservation.

Two techniques are used routinely for cryopreservation: *slow freezing* and *vitrification*. While the former, earlier technique is still used to cryopreserve embryos in some assisted reproduction laboratories, oocytes are cryopreserved exclusively using vitrification, since it was only with the introduction of this technique that the first consistently reproducible success with cryostorage of oocytes was achieved. With vitrification, cells are cooled rapidly and solidify to form a glass-like state.

Whether using slow freezing or vitrification, cryopreservation operates on the fundamental principle that to preserve cells at low temperatures (−196°C), it is essential to prevent ice crystal formation. This is achieved using two classes of cryoprotectants to protect the cells against cryodamage: *non-permeating* cryoprotectants, such as sucrose and trehalose, which act osmotically to dehydrate the cells, and *permeating* cryoprotectants, such as propanediol, glycerol and dimethyl sulphoxide (DMSO), which replace the water inside the cells. The major practical differences between slow freezing and vitrification are shown in Table 9.5.

With both cryopreservation techniques, embryos and oocytes are prepared for cryopreservation and thawed/warmed in a laminar flow hood using a sterile technique and appropriate witnessing. Oocytes/embryos are processed through a series of commercial preparations of appropriate reagents specific for the procedure, each maintained at

Table 9.5 Comparison of slow freezing and vitrification of embryos

	Slow freezing	Vitrification
Equipment	Programmed freeze machine	No machine required
Dehydration	Gradual	Rapid
Cryoprotectant concentration	Low (less toxic)	High (potentially toxic)
Temperature reduction	Gradual	Rapid
Maximum no. embryos processed together	Up to 20	1
Technical challenge	Low	High
Consistency of procedure	Consistent for each run of up to 20 embryos	Inter-operator and intra-operator variation between each embryo
Duration	~1.5 hours per freeze	~15 mins per embryo

temperatures between 37°C and room temperature, as stipulated by the manufacturer. It is important to use matching reagents for cryopreservation and the corresponding warming/thawing stages. Exposure to the different cryoprotectants in each one of the series of prepared reagents is time critical, particularly for vitrification where over-exposure to the relatively high concentration of cryoprotectants is toxic and some of the incubation steps are timed precisely, in seconds.

Oocytes and embryos are aspirated into straws (slow freezing) or placed onto one of a range of holding devices (vitrification) before cooling and storage in tanks (Dewars) of liquid nitrogen. The relatively large volume (0.25–0.5 mL) of straws used for slow freezing compared with the volume in which oocytes and embryos are held on vitrification devices (0.5–1 µL) means that vitrified material is at significantly greater risk of potentially fatal inadvertent uncontrolled warming, and care must be taken never to lift the vitrification devices from liquid nitrogen until intentional controlled warming for use in treatment takes place in the laboratory. In practice, this means that vitrified material requires significantly more storage space in Dewars than straws of an equivalent number of slow frozen embryos (Table 9.6).

For embryo cryopreservation, vitrification has become the method of choice in the majority of assisted reproduction laboratories worldwide and is widely held to yield higher success rates than slow freezing. Yet there is a lack of robust data from RCTs to support this [10]. Each of the two methods for embryo cryopreservation has distinct advantages and disadvantages (Table 9.6), the significance and impact of each of which may vary between different laboratories. Until one cryopreservation technique is

Table 9.6 Comparison of risks associated with slow freezing and vitrification

RISK	Slow freezing	Vitrification
Toxicity of cryoprotectant	+	+++
Osmotic stress	++	+++
Intracellular ice formation	+++	–
Accidental thawing	–	+++
Technology dependent	+++	–
Practitioner dependent	+/–	+++
Cost of consumables	+	+++
Storage space required	+	+++

shown definitively to yield better results than the other, the method of choice for any laboratory should be based on the technical ability and experience of staff in that laboratory, as well as on practical considerations relating to the facilities available, with the aim of providing the highest quality service, with maximum chance of successful outcome for patients.

9.13 Preimplantation Genetic Testing

Preimplantation genetic testing (PGT) is the umbrella term used to include all categories of testing the preimplantation embryo for genetic and/or chromosomal anomalies. Preimplantation genetic *diagnosis* (PGD), or PGT-M, refers to testing for a specific monogenic disorder. Preimplantation genetic *screening* (PGS) includes both PGT-A (preimplantation genetic testing

109

for aneuploidies) and PGT-SR (preimplantation genetic testing for chromosomal structural rearrangements). PGT entails the removal (biopsy) of cell(s) from the embryo and the analysis of their contents in the genetics laboratory. Advances in molecular genetics and the relative merits of techniques that are currently available for genetic analysis will not be considered here.

9.13.1 Preimplantation Genetic Diagnosis (PGT-M)

Preimplantation genetic diagnosis (PGT) is the earliest possible form of prenatal diagnosis for those who know they have a significant chance of a pregnancy carrying a serious genetic disorder, and who wish to avoid that risk. It is used to test for a specific mutation or chromosomal abnormality, including translocations, where the risk is known due to family history. PGD is used only when clinically indicated, after consideration of alternative reproductive options, in couples who have no option but to undergo some form of genetic testing of the conceptus if they are to have a child free of the disorder which they know the child is at risk of inheriting.

9.13.2 Preimplantation Genetic Screening (PGT-A and PGT-SR)

Preimplantation genetic screening (PGS) is used to test for aneuploidies where prospective parents do not have a known genetic abnormality but may be considered at risk, for example, due to maternal age, or following a previous aneuploid pregnancy. PGS is used for those who hope they may have an increased chance of achieving a pregnancy with assisted reproduction treatment if their embryos are screened for any sporadic, spontaneous chromosomal abnormalities, and if only those found to be free of such abnormalities are transferred. PGS is practised widely internationally but will remain a controversial technique until sufficient evidence demonstrates conclusively that it is more than theoretically beneficial. In light of this, PGS is not supported by NHS commissioning policy in the United Kingdom.

9.13.3 Preparation for Embryo Biopsy

The critical technique for PGT in the assisted reproduction laboratory is biopsy of cell(s) from the embryo, so that the biopsied material can be passed to the geneticists for analysis. Embryo biopsy is

carried out in a laminar flow hood, using sterile technique and appropriate witnessing, using the same micromanipulation rig as for ICSI (Figure 9.6).

9.13.4 Breaching the Zona Pellucida

Before it is possible to biopsy cells from the embryo, it is necessary to breach the zona pellucida. This may be done chemically (*zona drilling*), using acid Tyrode's solution which is relatively inexpensive but subject to inter-procedure and inter-operator variation, or mechanically, using a laser (*zona ablation*) which, though relatively expensive, uses a programmed laser to eliminate inter-procedure variation. For zona breaching, the embryo is placed in a 5- to 10-μL droplet of warmed (37°C) HEPES- or MOPS-buffered medium overlaid with mineral oil in a shallow petri dish (as used for ICSI). The dish is placed on the warm stage of the inverted phase microscope and held with a holding micropipette held in the left hand tool holder of the micromanipulators as for ICSI (Figure 9.6). For zona drilling, a small volume of acid Tyrode's solution, in a droplet adjacent to the droplet containing the oocyte, is aspirated into a drilling micropipette (8–12 μm internal diameter) held in the right hand tool holder that is used for the injection micropipette during ICSI (Figure 9.6). Acid Tyrode's solution is expelled carefully from the drilling micropipette onto a discrete area of the zona pellucida, while visualising the dissolution of the zona. As soon as the zona is breeched, the drilling micropipette is elevated from the dish and the embryo is released from the holding micropipette, rinsed in fresh warmed, pre-equilibrated culture medium to remove traces of acid Tyrode's solution, and returned to the incubator for culture until embryo biopsy.

For zona ablation, the embryo is held using a holding micropipette as for zona drilling and aligned appropriately before careful laser ablation using the appropriate ablation programme. After ablation, the embryo is released from the holding micropipette, placed in a dish of warmed, pre-equilibrated medium and returned to the incubator for culture until embryo biopsy.

9.13.5 Embryo Biopsy

Historically, PGT has been carried out using the genetic material from biopsied polar bodies, from biopsied cleavage stage blastomeres, and most recently from biopsied trophectoderm cells of blastocysts.

Polar body biopsy (Figure 9.12A):

- Biopsy of polar bodies from fertilised zygotes is performed on day 1 after oocyte retrieval and insemination.
- Polar bodies are the result of the two meiotic divisions; their chromosomal content is complementary to that of the oocyte after each meiotic division.
- Analysis of the polar bodies provides genetic analysis of the oocyte, not the embryo.
- Suitable only for testing for disorders of maternal origin.

Cleavage stage biopsy (Figure 9.12B):

- Biopsy of day 3 embryos is performed at the six- to eight-cell stage.
- Embryos may have undergone compaction when the blastomeres are tightly attached and difficult to remove.
- Necessitates pre-biopsy incubation in calcium-free medium to loosen attachments between blastomeres.
- Biopsied cleavage stage embryos may be left in culture for up to 2 days while awaiting results of genetic analysis.
- Will inevitably include biopsy of embryos that may not have the potential to continue to develop beyond the eight-cell stage.
- Safe to biopsy a maximum of two blastomeres (up to 25% of the embryo).
- Possible to carry out fresh embryo transfer on day 5.

Blastocyst stage biopsy (Figure 9.12C):

- This is the current method of choice.
- Zona breached on day 3/4 and embryos are returned to culture until day 5.
- Any embryos that form blastocysts will herniate trophectoderm through the breached zona as the blastocoel expands.

- Herniated trophectoderm cells can be excised using the laser, and biopsied cells collected for genetic analysis.
- Safe to biopsy 6–10 cells.
- Biopsied blastocysts must be cryopreserved while awaiting results of genetic analysis.
- There is less urgency in obtaining results of genetic tests.
- Only viable embryos that have developed into blastocysts are biopsied.
- Genetic tests can be processed in 'batches', introducing economy of scale into a costly process.
- Feasible only when carried out in conjunction with a successful cryopreservation service.

9.14 Summary

To optimise the chance of successful assisted reproduction treatment, consistent laboratory performance is critically important. Each of the numerous laboratory processes, from collection of the oocytes and preparation of the sperm for use in fertilisation in vitro, through embryo culture, assessment and selection for transfer, embryo biopsy for genetic testing, to the storage (cryopreservation) of gametes and embryos for use in later treatment, carries the inherent risk of damage, whether mechanical or through exposure to suboptimal conditions outside the body, with consequences for the chance of successful clinical outcome. While training, technical skills and consistent performance of all laboratory practitioners are vital pre-requisites for any clinical laboratory, the laboratory techniques for assisted reproduction are specific and unique. Procedures must be carried out meticulously, adhering to standard operating procedures (SOPs), with precise attention to detail. Strict adherence to guidelines issued by regulatory and professional bodies is necessary and essential in order to minimise risk and maximise performance, including the implementation of

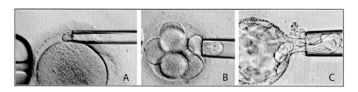

Figure 9.12 Strategies for embryo biopsy for PGT. (A) Polar body biopsy. (B) Cleavage stage biopsy. (C) Trophectoderm biopsy (blastocyst biopsy).

a Quality Management System (QMS) that ensures consistent, optimised performance, and facilitates risk and root cause analyses.

References

1. Association of Clinical Embryologists. Guidelines for good practice in clinical embryology laboratories. *Hum. Fertil.* 2012;**15**:174–89.

2. European Society for Human Reproduction and Embryology. Revised guidelines for good practice in IVF laboratories. 2015. Available at: www.eshre.eu/Guidelines-and-Legal/Guidelines/Revised-guidelines-for-good-practice-in-IVF-laboratories-(2015)

3. Mortimer ST, Mortimer D. *Quality and Risk Management in the IVF Laboratory.* Cambridge: Cambridge University Press; 2015.

4. Association of Biomedical Andrologists. Laboratory andrology guidelines for good practice version 3. *Hum Fertil.* 2012;**15**:156–73.

5. *WHO laboratory manual for the examination and processing of human semen,* 5th ed. Geneva: World Health Organization; 2010.

6. Verheyen G, Popovic-Todorovic B, Tournaye H. Processing and selection of surgically-retrieved sperm for ICSI: a review. *Basic Clin Androl.* 2017;**27**:6–15.

7. Jeve YB, Potdar N, Blower JA, Gelbaya T. Strategies to improve fertilisation rates with assisted conception: a systematic review. *Hum Fertil.* 2018;**21**:229–47.

8. On behalf of the British Fertility Society and the Association of Clinical Embryologists. How should we choose the 'best' embryo? A commentary. *Hum Fertil.* 2015;**18**:156–64.

9. On behalf of the Association of Clinical Embryologists (ACE) and the British Fertility Society (BFS). Elective single embryo transfer: an update to UK Best Practice Guidelines. *Hum Fertil.* 2015;**18**:165–83.

10. Rienzi L, Gracia C, Maggiulli R, LaBarbera AR, Kaser DJ, Ubaldi FM, et al. Oocyte, embryo and blastocyst cryopreservation in ART: systematic review and meta-analysis comparing slow-freezing versus vitrification to produce evidence for the development of global guidance. *Hum Reprod Update* 2017;**23**:139–55.

Chapter 10

Fertility Preservation

Maya Chetty and Richard A. Anderson

10.1 Introduction

- A broad range of malignant and benign conditions and their treatments can lead to the loss of future fertility in men and women, and in children of both sexes.
- Advances in cancer treatments have led to increased survival rates and therefore increasing numbers of young people living with the late effects of cancer treatments.
- Compromised fertility is the most common long-term side effect of cancer therapy and affects long-term wellbeing, relationships, and life decisions.
- The average age to have a first child has gradually increased and therefore increasing numbers of men and women have not completed their families when they are given a potentially fertility-damaging diagnosis.
- The endeavour to address this has grown into the new and rapidly developing field termed 'fertility preservation', although sperm cryopreservation for men has been available for many years.
- Fertility preservation encompasses a range of techniques to store material which can be used to achieve a pregnancy in the future, as well as techniques to minimise the damage caused by the fertility-damaging treatments.
- As this field involves a range of specialties and disciplines, generally with significant time pressures, effective communication and team-working are key to the success of fertility preservation programmes.
- Elective (often termed social) egg freezing is the freezing of eggs to enable women to delay the opportunity for pregnancy until a later time, for a non-medical indication. This uses the same techniques as used in oocyte cryopreservation for fertility preservation.

10.2 What Are the Indications for Fertility Preservation?

- Patients newly diagnosed with cancer, ideally at the pre-treatment stage, where there is a significant risk to later fertility. The most common indications for fertility preservation are breast cancer, testicular cancer and lymphoma. The risk of damage to fertility is mainly related to the treatment and not to the disease itself, although spermatogenesis is often significantly impaired at presentation due to the systemic effects of the cancer. This is less apparent in women. Alkylating chemotherapeutic agents and pelvic radiotherapy are particularly gonadotoxic (see Tables 10.1 and 10.2).
- Patients with benign medical or surgical conditions or undergoing medical or surgical treatment likely to compromise fertility. This includes cytotoxic agents for patients with rheumatological conditions, haematological conditions where treatment involves risk to fertility (e.g. haematopoietic stem cell transplant for haemoglobinopathy), inflammatory bowel disease, Turner syndrome and related chromosomal abnormalities, individuals with *FMRP1* mutations and patients with some metabolic diseases. There may also be some women facing treatment for endometriosis for whom consideration of fertility preservation is appropriate.
- The degree of risk to fertility that requires fertility preservation is rather subjective and should take into account the views of the patient, as well as a medical assessment of risk. More invasive and experimental procedures (e.g. ovarian tissue cryopreservation) may require a higher risk to fertility (estimated risk of loss >50%) than less invasive procedures such as semen cryopreservation. The time available, access to appropriate services

Table 10.1 Simplified risk of gonadotoxicity by treatment

	Females	Males
Higher risk	Whole abdominal or pelvic radiation (↑ doses, ↑age) Total body irradiation Alkylating chemotherapy (e.g. cyclophosphamide, busulphan) Protocols containing procarbazine (e.g. BEACOPP)	Testicular radiation (↑ doses) Pelvic radiation (↑ doses) Total body irradiation Alkylating chemotherapy (e.g. cyclophosphamide, busulphan) and cisplatin Protocols containing procarbazine (e.g. BEACOPP)
Lower risk	Non-alkylating chemotherapy	
Unknown risk	Taxanes Oxaliplatin Trastuzumab Imatinib	

For more details (females), see [1].

Table 10.2 Mechanism of gonadotoxicity of drugs used in cancer treatment

Drug type	Mechanism of Gonadotoxicity
Alkylating agents	Disrupt DNA synthesis and RNA transcription
Platinum analogue	Form crosslinks between DNA
Vinca alkaloid	Interfere with microtubule formation
Taxanes	Microtubule disruption
Anti-metabolites	Hinder DNA synthesis and transcription
Multikinase inhibitors	Unknown

and financial considerations will all also affect the decision. Criteria have been proposed as a basis for further development and validation (see Table 10.3).

- Transgender men and women. Both transwomen and transmen may want to store gametes prior to endocrine or surgical treatment. Though the effect of transgender endocrine treatment on fertility is considered reversible (for both spermatogenesis and folliculogenesis), once the treatment is initiated individuals may be very reluctant to take the prolonged break from it, with reversion to their dysphoric endocrine state, that would be required to restore fertility.

This list is not exhaustive and future research will define more clearly the indications and where the risk to future fertility is low.

10.3 Why Do Cancer Treatments Damage Fertility?

The primordial follicle pool, or ovarian reserve, is finite and complete before birth. It peaks at 18–22 weeks' gestation, with an average of 295,000 primordial follicles per ovary at birth, declining to 180,000 at 13 years. These are activated and used up across the reproductive life span. By 30 years of age, around 12% of the ovarian reserve remains, which declines to 3% by age 40 years. Only around 450 follicles will ovulate during a woman's reproductive lifetime, so the great majority of follicles undergo atresia, until insufficient follicles remain that can develop to later stages, resulting in the menopause at around 50 years. Age contributes to around 80% of the variation in ovarian reserve. Other determinants include genetic and lifestyle factors (stress, parity, basal metabolic index and smoking), the latter being thought to make a 3%–5% contribution to the age at menopause.

Cytotoxic chemotherapy and radiotherapy can cause a reduction in the number of ovarian follicles. Both specifically target DNA and dividing cells; thus growing follicles are important sites of damage, but primordial follicles may also be lost through either a direct effect or indirectly perhaps through increased initiation of growth.

Ovarian damage from chemotherapy and radiotherapy can occur via several mechanisms (Table 10.2) [3]:

1. Direct DNA damage to growing ovarian follicles causes apoptosis.
2. Direct damage to the ovarian stroma can result in fibrosis and hyalinisation of small blood vessels,

Table 10.3 The Edinburgh Selection Criteria for gonadal tissue cryopreservation

These were established with Ethical Committee review and approval, as these are experimental procedures and should be regarded as a starting point for future discussion, research and refinement.

Females	Age younger than 35 years
	No previous chemotherapy/radiotherapy if age >15 year at diagnosis, but mild, non-gonadotoxic chemotherapy is acceptable if <15 years
	A realistic chance of five-year survival
	A high risk of premature ovarian insufficiency (>50%)
	Informed consent (patient, parent where possible applicable)
	Negative HIV, syphilis and hepatitis serology
	Not pregnant and no existing children
Males	Age 0–16 years
	A high risk of infertility (>80%)
	Unable to produce a semen sample by masturbation
	No clinically significant pre-existing testicular disease (e.g. cryptorchidism)
	Informed consent (parent and, when possible, patient)
	Negative HIV, syphilis and hepatitis screening

From [2].

resulting in indirect follicle damage and probably compromising growth.

3. Both direct and indirect damage may alter the development of growing follicles and impair steroidogenesis.

4. The destruction of growing follicles causes loss of suppression of growth activation in primordial follicles, resulting in increased growth activation.

Radiation can also impact reproductive function through effects on the uterus, causing microvascular injury, endothelial damage and myometrial fibrosis resulting in poor uterine growth and distensibility resulting in miscarriage, preterm labour, low birth weight, stillbirth and postpartum haemorrhage. In contrast to the impact on ovarian function, the reproductive impact of uterine radiation is greater at a younger age, and pregnancy is of very high risk in those who have been exposed to uterine doses >45 Gy as adults or >25 Gy in childhood.

In males both chemotherapy and radiation therapy can result in germ cell depletion with the development of oligo- or azoospermia. The type of drug (particularly the alkylating agents), duration of treatment, intensity of treatment and drug combination are major variables in determining the extent and duration of testicular injury. Different drugs disrupt spermatogenesis in different ways (see Table 10.2). Spermatogonia proliferate rapidly and so represent the most sensitive target for cytotoxic agents although the less active stem cell pool may also be depleted (see Figure 10.1). Recovery of sperm production after a cytotoxic therapy depends on the survival and ability

of mitotically quiescent stem spermatogonia to transform into actively dividing stem and differentiating spermatogonia.

The likelihood of infertility after radiation of the testes depends on the dose to the testes, shielding and fractionation. The Leydig cells (responsible for testosterone production) are less sensitive to the effects of radiation, with damage occurring at 20 Gy in prepubescent males compared with 30 Gy in mature males.

In both males and females radiotherapy can also adversely affect reproductive function through damage to the hypothalamus and pituitary.

For both men and women, loss of fertility is often temporary, provided a sufficient testicular population of spermatogonial stem cells or ovarian supply of primordial follicles remains.

10.4 Who Should Be Offered Fertility Preservation?

Within the United Kingdom, the National Institute for Health and Care Excellence (NICE) (2013) guidance recommends that fertility preservation (sperm or oocyte/embryo cryopreservation) should be offered where a threat exists from oncological treatments or illnesses that compromise fertility [4]. The British Fertility Society has also produced clear guidelines for fertility preservation in adult women, as have other organisations including the American Society for Clinical Oncology [1, 5]. Importantly, the NICE document sets out a number of factors that should be taken

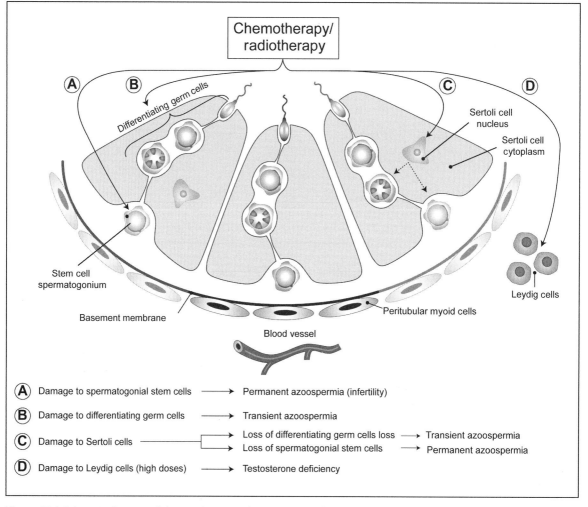

Figure 10.1 Schematic showing cellular site of action and consequences of chemo- and radiotherapy in males.

into account when considering fertility preservation, including the diagnosis, treatment plan, expected outcome of subsequent fertility treatment and viability of stored/post-thawed material. In addition, for females, it is highlighted that they need to be fit enough and that there is time available to undergo ovarian stimulation and egg collection, and that this will not worsen their condition. Given the strict criteria for access to NHS IVF programmes, NICE also emphasises that the eligibility criteria applied for access to funded infertility treatment/IVF should not be applied. To ensure that fertility preservation is always discussed with patients when it needs to be, it needs to be considered for all patients and then discussed as early as possible in their treatment pathway in the cases where it is appropriate to do so.

10.5 Assessment of the Patient Prior to Fertility Preservation

This can be considered in terms of the patient him/herself ('intrinsic' issues) and those factors that the patient is going to be exposed to ('extrinsic' issues) (see Box 10.1).

- Intrinsic factors include their general health status (e.g. coagulopathy, mediastinal mass that may complicate anaesthesia, pelvic tumour), psychological state, age, consideration of her ovarian reserve or current spermatogenesis for women and men respectively and pubertal status in adolescents.
- Extrinsic factors largely hinge on the proposed treatment (table of gonadotoxic therapy). This

Box 10.1 Risk Assessment: Intrinsic and Extrinsic Factors That Should Be Taken into Account When Considering Fertility Preservation Strategies

Intrinsic Factors

Health status of the patient

Psychosocial factors

Consent (patient/parent)

Assessment of pubertal status

Assessment of ovarian reserve (females) or spermatogenesis (males)

Extrinsic Factors

Nature of predicted treatment (high/medium/low/uncertain risk)

Time available

Expertise/technical options available

may be clear, and can be categorised as low, medium or high risk to fertility. However, it may be that staging investigations or diagnostic tests are incomplete. A significant complicating factor is also the risk of recurrence, which will generally entail treatment with much higher risk to fertility.

10.6 What Storage Options Are Available for Males?

- Sperm cryopreservation has been widely available since the 1970s and is the most effective way of preserving male fertility. Samples are most commonly produced by masturbation, though if this is not possible vibratory stimulation devices, electro-ejaculation or surgical sperm retrieval techniques can be used. Samples are diluted with cryoprotectant and stored in nitrogen vapour.
- The quality does not deteriorate over time, and cryopreserved sperm have been used in successful fertility treatment after 40 years of cryopreservation. However, sperm are inevitably damaged by the freeze–thaw process.
- Usage can be either in intrauterine insemination or in vitro fertilisation (IVF)/intracytoplasmic sperm injection (ICSI), depending on the quality and quantity of the sperm available, as well as taking female factors into account.
- The use of cryopreserved sperm is small: only around 10% of sperm samples stored actually go on to be used in fertility treatments. This may be because the man's fertility was not lost, his death or personal circumstances.

- Mature sperm begin to appear in the ejaculate during puberty and sperm cryopreservation is potentially feasible in those older than 13 years, and earlier in some. Assessment and discussion in boys at these ages raises specific challenges, including parental involvement. There are currently no established fertility preservation options for pre-pubertal males. Experimental approaches include removing testicular tissue for cryostorage, with the possibility of subsequent re-transplantation or in vitro maturation of germ cells. While there are centres in the United Kingdom and elsewhere offering prepubertal testicular cryostorage, there are no cases in which tissue has been replaced or sperm cells matured.

10.7 What Storage Options Are Available for Females?

Storage options for post-pubertal/adult women are egg or embryo cryopreservation, or ovarian tissue cryopreservation (see Figure 10.2). Embryo cryopreservation is the most established, being part of IVF treatment for decades. Historically, oocyte cryopreservation has been problematic, with slow freezing (the method until recently also used for embryo cryopreservation) resulting in very low success rates. The development of oocyte vitrification in the early years of this century enabled a revolution in oocyte cryopreservation–suddenly cryopreserved oocytes had very similar developmental competence to fresh oocytes. While of huge benefit for fertility preservation, this has also led to the development of 'egg banks' for

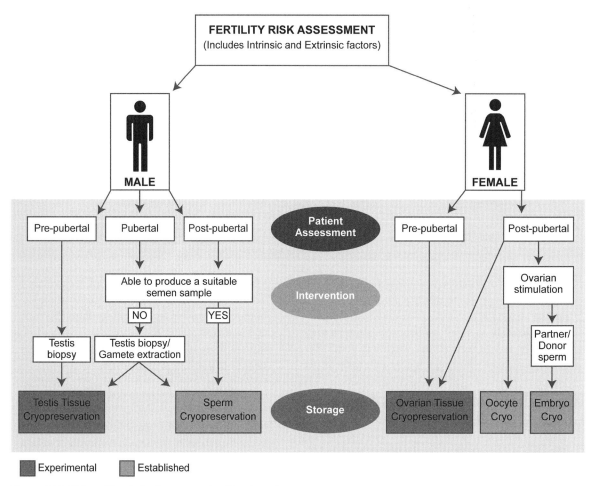

Figure 10.2 Male and female fertility preservation: Flowchart of options.

donation purposes and has underpinned the expansion of elective egg freezing.

Both embryo and oocyte cryopreservation are based on ovarian stimulation, as used for IVF. The specific needs of fertility preservation patients (notably avoidance of delay in starting treatment) have led to the development of novel approaches, most importantly 'random start' protocols (see Figure 10.3). These make use of the recognition that follicles can be successfully stimulated to grow at all stages of the menstrual cycle, including the luteal phase, and as oocytes or embryos will be frozen, the state of the endometrium is irrelevant. Gonadotropin-releasing hormone (GnRH) antagonist-based protocols avoid the need for lengthy downregulation, a key feature of traditional protocols and the use of GnRH agonist as trigger instead of human chorionic gonadotropin reduces the risk of ovarian hyperstimulation syndrome (OHSS).

The risks of ovarian stimulation include OHSS (reduced but not avoided completely with the use of a GnRH antagonist cycle and a GnRH agonist trigger), the anaesthetic and operative risks of an egg collection and the risks of disseminating pelvic malignancy. Anti-oestrogens (e.g. letrozole or tamoxifen) can be used during ovarian stimulation in women with oestrogen-sensitive tumours, for example, in some breast cancers, and similarly can also be used in transmen to minimise oestrogen exposure.

Embryo Cryopreservation

- Embryo cryopreservation is the most established method of female fertility preservation. The process involves controlled ovarian stimulation, egg collection, fertilisation with sperm and then cryopreservation of embryos for future use. This

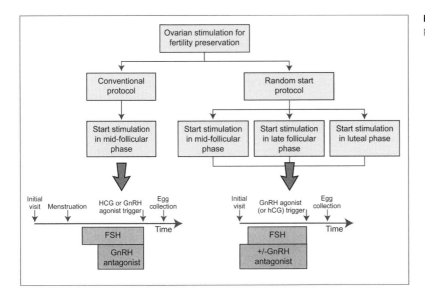

Figure 10.3 Ovarian stimulation protocols for fertility preservation.

process takes approximately 2–3 weeks from start to egg collection and chemotherapy can be started after 48 hours.

- If a partner's sperm has been used, his consent is required in the future for the embryos to be utilised. It is essential that this information is clearly conveyed to both partners, and that the woman in particular understands the implications of her partner withdrawing consent.

- Embryos are most effectively stored at the blastocyst stage. However, if future genetic testing may be required (e.g. preimplantation genetic testing for *BRCA* gene mutations in patients with breast cancer) it may be beneficial to store at an earlier stage.

- Using the embryos requires the preparation of the endometrium in a natural or artificial thaw cycle, and an embryo transfer. Approximately 90% of good quality blastocysts survive the thawing process and live birth rates are approximately 35% per good quality blastocyst transferred.

Oocyte Cryopreservation ('Egg Freezing')
- Oocyte cryopreservation has become a useful alternative to embryo cryopreservation since the development of oocyte vitrification ('flash-freezing'). This newer technique is much more effective than the older slow-freezing technique, and vitrified oocytes have

a developmental potential very similar to that of fresh oocytes.

- The same processes are used as in embryo cryopreservation (controlled ovarian stimulation and egg collection), but oocytes are not inseminated and so their future use does not require the consent of the partner who provided the sperm.

- Ninety to ninety-five per cent of vitrified oocytes survive the thawing process and success rates are approximately 6% per thawed oocyte. In cumulative terms, if a woman under 35 years old stores 15 mature eggs she has more than an 80% chance of at least one live birth.

Ovarian Tissue Cryopreservation
- Ovarian tissue cryopreservation (OTC) is increasingly regarded as no longer experimental in adult women but is the only option for pre-pubertal girls. It is an option for post-pubertal females, particularly where there is inadequate time to complete ovarian stimulation. Ovarian cortex (as this is where primordial follicles are located) is harvested laparoscopically either by unilateral oophorectomy or by removal of ovarian cortex, and slow frozen in small pieces.

- Tissue is re-implanted by transplanting thawed pieces of tissue into either the medullary portion of the remaining ovary or a nearby peritoneal pocket.

Table 10.4 Advantages and disadvantages of OTC as compared with oocyte/embryo cryopreservation

Ovarian tissue cryopreservation	Oocyte/embryo cryopreservation
Advantages	
Quicker process (depending on access to theatre)	Widely available
Potential restoration of endocrine function	Higher chance of live birth
Potential for natural conception	Less invasive
Possible in pre-pubertal girls	
Disadvantages	
More invasive (two laparoscopies required)	Slower process so may delay start of chemotherapy
Anaesthetic risks (two general anaesthetics required)	Supraphysiological hormone levels
Potential for tissue contamination with micrometastatic disease	Requires assisted reproduction clinic for use of stored materials
Smaller chance of live birth	and conception

- Resumption of normal menstrual cycles has been reported in more than 90% of patients within 4–9 months of after transplantation. The restoration of sex steroid production is a benefit of ovarian tissue replacement over egg/embryo fertility preservation.
- The live birth rate is approximately 25%, and more than 100 live births have been achieved worldwide with this technique. At present only one birth has been achieved from tissue stored in adolescence (early puberty) and one from tissue obtained in childhood (pre-puberty): both of these cases were for haematological disease rather than cancer. The duration of graft function has varied widely from a few months to more than 10 years: at present this appears to be unpredictable.
- There is a risk of reintroduction of the original malignancy. This risk is high in leukaemia, where there are circulating malignant cells. Careful histology and consideration of the use of molecular markers is essential to minimise this risk in all cases.
- OTC is still not an established treatment and is offered only by the small number of units who have the relevant expertise, protocols and licensing.

10.8 What Are the Pregnancy Outcomes in Cancer Survivors?

Large prospective studies have shown no increase in abnormalities in children conceived using cryopreserved sperm, oocytes or embryos.

Abdomino-pelvic radiotherapy can cause uterine damage which reduces the chance of implantation, increases the risk of miscarriage, placental dysfunction and preterm birth. Where significant uterine damage has occurred, surrogacy should be considered.

10.9 Ethical and Legal Issues

10.9.1 Surgical Sperm Retrieval

Surgical sperm retrieval (SSR) can be performed as an emergency to collect sperm from someone who is unable to give their consent to storage, but only if the person is likely to regain the capacity to consent at some point in the future. Gametes from a person who has died (including cases of brain stem death) cannot be stored or used without that person's written consent. Unlike organs and other tissues, no one can give consent on behalf of a gamete provider.

10.9.2 Storage

The standard maximum storage period for gametes or embryos, according to the Human Fertilisation and Embryology (HFE) Act (1990) and 2009 regulations, is ten years. This can be extended to a maximum of 55 years if the person who stored the gametes or one of the people whose gametes was used to create the embryos is prematurely infertile or likely to become so. Extension of storage beyond 10 years requires the written consent of the relevant person(s) and a written statement from a medical practitioner. People storing gametes or embryos must be informed of these statutory storage limits and understand that if they do not meet the criteria for premature infertility, storage cannot be extended beyond 10 years. Ovarian tissue cryostorage is licensed by the Human Tissue Authority, not the Human Fertilisation and Embryology Authority; thus these limitations do not (at present) apply.

10.9.3 Posthumous Use

While a patient can give consent to the posthumous storage and use of their gametes, storage and use is possible only for the duration of their consent. A partner can be nominated to use the gametes or embryos posthumously but they cannot be left to parents or anyone else to decide in the future who can use them.

10.9.4 Surrogacy

Women with gynaecological malignancies and trans males undergoing gender reassignment may wish to store gametes or embryos prior to having a hysterectomy. It therefore needs to be discussed that, unless they are in a same-sex relationship, they will require a surrogate to carry a pregnancy for them in the future. Surrogacy is a legally complex area and the current UK law is under review. Commercial surrogacy arrangements are illegal in the United Kingdom but 'reasonable expenses' can be paid and can be very high. The surrogate mother is the legal mother at birth and then the intended parents apply to the family court for a parental order. A parental order will make both of the intended parents the legal parents and permanently extinguish the surrogate's legal motherhood. Anyone considering using a surrogate should be advised to seek independent legal advice.

10.9.5 Counselling

Counselling from a trained counsellor should be offered both prior to fertility preservation and prior to the use of stored material. This is to both aid with decision making and to provide psychological support.

10.10 What Preventative Options Are Available for Women?

10.10.1 Ovarian Transposition

To protect the ovaries from radiation injury they can be surgically moved out of the radiation field. This technique is called ovarian transposition or suspension and can be useful prior to radiotherapy for cervical, rectal and colon cancer, pelvic Hodgkin's lymphoma and Ewing's sarcoma. The procedure is usually performed laparoscopically and involves transection of the ovarian ligament and mobilisation of the ovary. The ovarian blood supply is maintained through the infundibulopelvic ligament. Fallopian tubes should not be transected so that the potential for natural conception is retained. The ovaries can be marked with metallic clips so that they are identifiable

radiologically. There is little good quality evidence as to the effectiveness of ovarian transposition.

10.10.2 Ovarian Shielding

External shielding and intensity-modulated radiation therapy have been used to try and minimize radiation damage to the ovaries but have not been found to be effective. Proton therapy may offer more targeted pelvic radiotherapy in the future.

10.10.3 Ovarian Suppression

Suppression of ovarian function with GnRH agonists prior to and during chemotherapy has been shown to significantly reduce the risk of premature ovarian failure in pre-menopausal women with early breast cancer. [6]. Whether this translates into a greater opportunity for conception, or longer-term benefits of endocrine ovarian function, remains unclear. The mechanism of this 'ovarian protection' is not entirely understood. Ovarian suppression will reduce ovarian blood flow, which may reduce the amount of chemotherapy agents that the ovary is exposed to. Another theory is that the GnRH agonist prevents the rise in luteinizing hormone and follicle-stimulating hormone caused by the destruction of growing follicles by chemotherapy drugs which stimulates more follicles to enter the maturation pathway, making them more susceptible to the damaging effects of the chemotherapy.

10.10.4 Fertility Sparing Surgery

Fertility-sparing surgery is used in gynaecological cancers with the aim of retaining fertility whilst achieving outcomes that are not inferior to more extensive conventional surgery. Radical trachelectomy is a well-established fertility sparing option for young women with early stage cervical carcinoma. In borderline ovarian tumours there is concern about the effect of ovarian stimulation and the risk of microscopic seeding of tumour at egg collection after cystectomy.

10.11 What Preventative Options Are Available for Men?

There are currently no recommended approaches to protect spermatogenesis in male patients undergoing chemotherapy. Testicular shielding can minimise the testicular damage caused by radiotherapy.

10.12 What Other Options Are Available?

When fertility preservation is discussed alternatives should also be explained and considered. These include the possibility of gamete donation, adoption and life without children. Donor sperm is widely available in the United Kingdom and can be used for insemination treatment or IVF. Donor eggs are less easily accessible and so many people choose to go overseas where there are large and very successful egg donation programmes. In UK law donors cannot donate anonymously. Children resulting from donor gametes or embryos have the right to non-identifying information about the donor from the age of 16 and identifying information from the age of 18.

References

1. Loren AW, Mangu PB, Beck LN, et al. Fertility preservation for patients with cancer: American Society of Clinical Oncology clinical practice guideline update. *J Clin Oncol*, 2013; **31**: 2500–10.

2. Anderson RA, Mitchell RT, Kelsey TW, Spears N, Telfer EE and Wallace WH. Cancer treatment and gonadal function: experimental and established strategies for fertility preservation in children and young adults. *Lancet Diabetes Endocrinol*, 2015;3:556–67.

3. Jayasinghe YL, W. Wallace WHB and Anderson RA. Ovarian function, fertility and reproductive lifespan in cancer patients. *Expert Rev Endocrinol Metab*, 2018;**13**:3, 125–36, DOI: 10.1080/17446651.2018.1455498.

4. National Institute for Clinical Excellence. Fertility: assessment and treatment for people with fertility problems (2013) http://publicationsniceorguk/fertility-cg156

5. Yasmin E, Balachandren N, Davies MC, et al. Fertility preservation for medical reasons in girls and women: British fertility society policy and practice guideline. *Hum Fertil*, 2018 21:3–26.

6. Lambertini M, Moore HCF, Leonard RCF, et al. Gonadotropin-releasing hormone agonists during chemotherapy for preservation of ovarian function and fertility in premenopausal patients with early breast cancer: A systematic review and meta-analysis of individual patient-level data. *J Clin Oncol*, 2018; **36**: 1981–90.

Further Reading

Donnez J, Dolmans MM Fertility preservation in women. *N Engl J Med*, 2017;**377**:1657–65.

RCOG Pregnancy and Breast Cancer Green–top Guideline No. 12 (2011). www.rcog.org.uk/globalassets/documents/guidelines/gtg_12.pdf

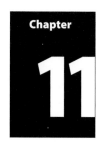

Third-Party Reproduction
Psychosocial Aspects in Infertility Practice

Petra Nordqvist, Petra Thorn and Jacky Boivin

11.1 Third-Party Reproduction and the Human Fertilisation Embryology Authority Code of Practice

As described earlier, third-party reproduction refers to fertility care that involves medically assisted reproduction using gametes or embryos that have been donated or provided by a third person (donor) to enable an individual or couple (intended parents) to become parents. It can also refer to the use of surrogacy, where a woman (surrogate) other than the intended parent carries the pregnancy.

The Human Fertilisation Embryology Authority (HFEA) Code of Practice (9th edition, 2019) helps clinics comply with the legal requirements to prepare patients for treatment, as set out in the Human Fertilisation and Embryology Act 1990. According to this code, the person responsible, often the clinician, should have sufficient knowledge of all aspects of the infertility clinic to supervise its activities properly including its psychosocial aspects. Furthermore, the Code provides very clear guidance that for all treatments, including third-party reproduction, centres must ensure that patients are well prepared prior to treatment for all aspects of treatment Section 4.1, HFEA). This preparation makes it mandatory for the patient, donor, surrogate and their partners to be provided with information as is relevant for their treatment option (see [1] for details of information provision), be given a suitable opportunity to have a discussion about the implications of taking the proposed steps and be offered the opportunity to be supported through counselling. The code also makes clear that patients should be supported throughout treatment and provides two mechanisms by which this could be achieved: patient support that all members of staff are expected to provide and specialised psychosocial counselling that only qualified infertility counsellors can provide. Quality indicators are used to assess current and expected performance regarding these two components of psychosocial support (i.e. benchmarks for quality). In the 9th edition, for the first time, there is a clearly defined section about expectations for patient support.

In this chapter we present a brief overview of the psychosocial aspects of providing fertility treatment, especially as is relevant to third-party reproduction (see HFEA Code of Practice for more in-depth information).

11.2 HFEA Patient Support Policy and Counselling Requirements

11.2.1 Patient Support

Fertility clinics in the United Kingdom are required to develop a Patient Support Policy (see Box 11.1) that outlines how the Centre providing treatment ensures that patients, donors and their partners receive appropriate psychosocial support before, during and after treatment from all staff they encounter. This psychosocial support is considered to be patient-centred care (PCC), which should be defined within clinic policy. PCC consists in providing care that is ' . . . respectful of and responsive to individual patient preferences, needs, and values and ensuring that patient values guide all clinical decisions" [2, p. 6]. In fertility care, 11 PCC dimensions have been identified as important to patients (e.g. availability of specialised infertility staff, continuity of care during treatment, clear communication, high patient involvement and emotional support). Guidelines based on systematic review of available evidence exist to help staff develop these policies [1]. Quality indicators for patient support services are not yet developed because this is a new component of the HFEA Code of Practice. However, at minimum it is expected it will involve patient satisfaction.

Box 11.1 Key Points of the HFEA Code of Practice 9th edition (2019) Patient Support Policy

HFEA Code of Practice 9th edition (2019) stipulates that Centre's **Patient Support Policy** must outline the

- Patient-centred care at the clinic (what it is, role of each staff in delivering it)
- The internal and external resources available to patients (information, peer-to-peer support, events, interventions customised to treatments and different user groups)
- Strategy for communication with patients
- Annual program of staff training for different aspects of patient support (tailored to staff roles)
- Data collection methods for quality indicators, relevant monitoring, feedback and quality improvement (e.g., user satisfaction with support, offer of counselling, provision of healthy lifestyle advice)

Centre management should ensure that staff members who are in contact with patients, and donors and their partners (where applicable):

- Follow the 'patient support policy'
- Are prepared to offer appropriate emotional support to people suffering distress
- Understand and can explain the role of counselling
- Know when and how to refer people to the centre's qualified infertility counsellor
- Are sensitive to any ethnic, religious, societal, cultural or other factors that may influence the kind of support which is appropriate for an individual

---

11.2.2 Preparation for and Counselling Prior to Treatment

The law requires that all patients be prepared for treatment, and that preparation involves providing information (see [1] for information required for informed consent), discussing implications of treatment choices and the offer of counselling.

The law states (for counselling): 'A woman shall not be provided with treatment ... unless she or any man or woman who is to be treated together with her have been given a suitable opportunity to receive proper counselling ... ' [1], p. 26. The law makes very clear that the offer of counselling is mandatory, and the groups to whom it should be offered, namely the individuals considering any treatment that:

- Uses donated gametes or embryos (including mitochondrial donation)
- Creates embryos in vitro
- Requires the storage of gametes (though some exceptions)
- Involves donation of gametes or embryos or mitochondrial (for treatment of others, research or training or any reason)
- Requires the consent for a man (in heterosexual couples) or woman (in lesbian couples) to be treated as the legal parent of any child as a result of a woman's treatment

11.2.3 Types of Counselling

The HFEA Act (1990) gives only minimal information about what counselling should comprise and does not stipulate who should provide that counselling. As a result, there is potential for confusion in the HFEA Code of Practice about the nature and provider of counselling. The HFEA Code of Practice recognises potential for confusion over the term counselling, and therefore explicitly differentiates 'proper counselling' in two ways. One type of counselling described in the law and code of practice is counselling about the implications of using particular treatment options (' ... proper counselling about the implications of her being provided with that treatment ... ' [1], p. 26). This form of counselling is referred to as 'discussion of implications' in the new Code of Practice ([1], Section 4.2, p. 34). The second form of counselling is counselling directed specifically at providing specialised psychosocial care related to infertility and fertility care. This form of counselling (referred to as 'infertility counselling', Section 2.14, p. 22) is mentioned in the Code of Practice but not in the law. The HFEA Code of Practice explicitly states that this type of infertility (psychosocial) counselling should be differentiated from the counsel provided in activities that other staff do, namely discussions about the implications of treatment; assessment of a person's suitability to receive fertility care, to store

---

Box 11.2 Key Points of the Offer of Infertility Counselling

According to the HFEA the **offer of infertility counselling** is mandatory for all fertility care, including third-party reproduction. The offer and uptake (or not) of counselling should be documented.

The HFEA requires that the offer of infertility counselling be made so as to optimise the opportunity for patients to take it up. It should be

- Offered to all patients, donors, surrogates and their partners where it is legally recommended to do so (schedule 3ZA), with both members of a couple encouraged to attend together
- Made as accessible as possible for all (i.e., patients, donors and surrogates), including to those having previously donated or received treatment
- Described as a routine part of the treatment pathway
- Offered prior to treatment with sufficient time for people to consider and take up the offer before consent
- Repeated throughout treatment, donation or storage processes and routinely following adverse events and/or unsuccessful outcomes
- Offered separately to surrogates and intended parents
- Made with written information about the counsellor (name, availability, accessibility)

Only qualified counsellors with specialist competence in infertility can offer psychosocial counselling. The counsellor may be staff at the centre or external to it (depending on patient preference). Several organisations provide accreditation of counsellors in the United Kingdom.

---

or donate their gametes or embryos (including mitochondrial donation); and the provision of information for informed consent or the supportive relationship expected from clinical staff towards their patient (or donors) (Section 3.7).

It is important to know the distinction between these two forms of counselling because the providers are different. Clinic staff with the appropriate skills, knowledge and experience of the specified treatment can discuss the implications of treatment with patients but only 'infertility counsellors' specialised in providing psychosocial care can provide 'infertility counselling'. In previous codes of practice (e.g. 7th edition) these two forms of counselling were sometimes confused by the use of the generic term 'implications counselling' to refer to discussions about implications.

Aside from these main types, specialist counselling may be recommended if required (e.g. genetic counselling, counselling for mitochondrial donation, counselling for oncology patients).

Doctors should become knowledgeable about infertility counselling and how to make an optimal offer of counselling (see Box 11.2). Centres are required to report as a quality indicator the number of patients offered and taking up, or declining, infertility counselling.

11.3 Psychosocial Issues in Third-Party Reproduction

The HFEA prefers that patients discuss with infertility counsellors the implications of their treatment options and choices (Section 20.9, HFEA Code of Practice) because such discussions often raise emotional and psychosocial issues, especially in the case of third-party reproduction. If the patient decides not to take up the offer of counselling then the person responsible should ensure the patient has the opportunity to discuss implications of the treatment with another member of staff with sufficient skill, knowledge and experience. In third-party reproduction, discussion about the implications of treatment with donated material (gametes, mitochondria) should be done separately from discussion about the implications of treatment in general. Detailed and clearly presented written information and guidance should be provided to support the discussion about implications, at a level of complexity tailored to the needs of those receiving the information. The centre should actively probe understanding of all parties and encourage individuals to ask questions. Treatment should be provided only when the centre is satisfied that all parties understand all aspects of the arrangement and are entering into the arrangement freely and voluntarily.

11.3.1 Overview of Implication Discussion (Embedded or Not in Infertility Counselling)

The psychological issues explored prior to treatment will differ according to the treatment option and relevance of issues to them as a specific patient group (patient, donor, surrogate, partner). This psychological discussion will often involve valuing and deliberating the pros and cons of the different options available to patients. The implication discussion also involves discussion of legal issues. Consent and legal parenthood are complex processes that involve consideration of the partnership status (married, civil partner), potential future events (death) and multiple perspectives (patients, donors, partners, child). Clinics differ in regards to who is authorised to take consent. Discussion of legal issues regarding being a donor or a surrogate or the use of donated gametes is not possible here but professionals should be aware that discussion of these very complex issues and the legal preparatory work related to them (such as surrogacy, treatment of same-sex couples, etc.) will require specialised staff (e.g. solicitors) (see HFEA Code of Practice for more information).

The implication discussion is confidential. However, patients need to be informed in advance that staff (including infertility counsellors) have a duty of care and may need to disclose any information as permitted by law that gives rise to concerns about the suitability of a person to donate gametes, whether a surrogate or a prospective parent (i.e. welfare of the child).

11.3.2 Psychosocial Issues in Third-Party Reproduction

The implication discussion needs to consider the range of psychosocial issues to emerge throughout the process of third-party reproduction (from initial decision-making to future life with children). Psychosocial issues need to be addressed in advance of consenting, before irrevocable events have taken place. It should be noted that the specific issues to emerge during the implication discussion(s) can apply to all intended parents or to only specific groups (e.g. heterosexual couples, lesbians). Tables 11.1 and 11.2 present some of the issues to emerge.

11.3.2.1 The Decision to Use Third-Party Conception

When patients discuss the implications of using third-party reproduction they often revisit how they came to this decision, and what they perceive to be the implications to themselves and their current and future family (see Table 11.1). Most people

Table 11.1 Topics considered in the decision to use third-party reproduction

Issues typically addressed by most intended parents using donated gametes
Acknowledging the emotional burden of involuntary childlessness, infertility and failed treatment cycles (if applicable)
Supporting mourning of fertility and the fact that there may not be a genetic relation between the child and (both) parents; exploring the consequences of the possible (genetic) asymmetry in the parent–child relationship between parents
Exploring beliefs and values attached to third-party reproduction (incl. type of donation such as open/known or anonymous donation, double donation, etc.) and its alternatives (e.g. adoption, fostering, remaining childless)
Exploring the current personal and family situation as well as the short- and long-term implications of using donated gametes/surrogacy (for example the possibility that the wider family may not understand the use of third-party reproduction, potential reactions of grandparents to a non-genetic grandchild, potential stigma towards the child; the risk of the surrogate not wishing to relinquish the baby or sign the parental order; impact of ethnicity and race on perceptions of and reactions to third-party reproduction)
Providing medical, legal and financial information (typical treatment procedures, regulations regarding legal parenthood, the number of offspring per donor documentation of donor records, right of the child to access these, etc.)
Supporting decision-making (type of donor, type of surrogate)
Informing about the implications of treatment (e.g. medical issues such as the limitations of donor screening in avoiding transmissible conditions and psychosocial issues such as how and when to disclose the nature of conception to the child and significant others, the possibility of meeting the donor/surrogate and/or [half-]siblings)
Reviewing (and providing) support needs during treatment, as patients may experience treatment failures
Exploring (and providing) ongoing support needs after the birth of the child (including supporting disclosure, facilitating contact between offspring (and family) and donor/surrogate (and family); helping on issues related to egg and sperm imported from other countries (where the 10 family limit does not apply); discussing future child use of direct-to-consumer DNA testing.

See ref. [2].

Table 11.2 Specific patient needs among heterosexual couples, lesbian couples and single women (additional to those listed in Table 11.1)

Specific issues experienced by most common user groups of third-party reproduction		
Heterosexual couples	**Lesbian couples**	**Single women**
• Feelings of grief and loss about infertility and not having a genetically related child together • Feelings of failure due to the need to use donated gametes; threat to femininity and masculinity • Negative reaction to partner being pregnant with the sperm of an unknown man • Negative reaction to partner who can become a genetic parent	• Decision-making about who will be the gestating parent • Understanding that the role and identity of the social or non-genetic parent is often not culturally, socially and legally well recognised or acknowledged • Children can face double stigma (use of donated gametes and sexual orientation of parent) • Wider family may have unfavourable view of lesbian or gay family constellations	• Feelings of sadness about not having a family with a partner, which is often the preferred choice • Mixed feelings about the use donated gametes • Children can face double stigma (use of donated gametes and solo status of parent) • Wider family may lack understanding of motives to be a solo parent or have unfavourable view of it

See refs. [2–5].

come to the decision to use third-party reproduction after a significant period of deliberation (sometimes years). It is a significant decision for many reasons but especially because in most societies there is a very strong importance attached to the genetic connectedness of family. This revisiting is an important aspect of understanding that could affect all aspects of the patients' experience of third-party reproduction.

In addition to the issues that most intended parents experience, it is important to recognise that different patient groups also have needs, feelings and experiences specific to them (see Table 11.2). The diversity of patients accessing third-party reproduction is considerable and include both single people (cisgender men and women, trans and intersex individuals) and different couple constellations (heterosexual, gay and lesbian couples, couples where one or both partners are trans or intersex). Within these groups, people seek access to third-party reproduction because of issues relating to infertility, but also as a chosen route to parenthood (e.g. lesbian couples). The most commonly treated patient groups in the United Kingdom, according to HFEA statistics (Human Fertilisation and Embryology Authority, 2018 Fertility Treatment 2014–2016: Trends and Figures), are heterosexual couples, lesbian couples and single women. However, it is important that clinicians also understand the specific needs and experiences of trans and intersex individuals, gay couples and single men.

11.3.2.2 Choosing the Donor and Thinking Through the Future Relationship with Him or Her

It is important for people considering third-party reproduction to discuss which donor to choose. This can involve consideration of physical characteristics but also the type of and level of contact and closeness with an identifiable donor that the intended parent(s) and the donor desire. In discussing such issues patients may request and make use of non-identifying the information (e.g. pen portraits) donors provide about themselves (interests, likes and dislikes, approaches to life and educational background). Patients have a right to request this information at any stage of treatment.

It is established practice among clinicians and parents to choose a donor who resembles the couple, particularly in physical features and ethnicity. Although a common approach, it can be problematic because it reinforces the idea of race/ethnicity being an inheritable characteristic.

Since 1 April 2005, anonymous donation and the use of non-traceable imported gametes is no longer permitted in the United Kingdom. All treatments with donated gametes or embryos in the United Kingdom use an identity-release framework whereby the child upon request can receive identifiable information (name, address) about the donor at the age of 18 years. In addition to this, some parents choose to use a known identified donor. A known donor is one known to the family (e.g. a sister, friend) before the start of treatment or a contact the intended parent(s) purposefully developed for donating, for example, via online communities. It is worth noting that among lesbian and gay communities especially, known donation has been informally practiced for a long time.

Another key area of consideration (and decision) is the level of contact and closeness between the donor and the parents and child. The child cannot know that they have been conceived with donated gametes or embryo unless the parent(s) disclose this information to them (or they inadvertently discover it). UK law does not require parents to tell their child but the HFEA Code of Practice and 2008 Act (1) recommends that parents should disclose this information to any resulting child at an early age. This information enables the child to grow up in full knowledge of their genetic origins and, in due course, to realise their right to seek and initiate contact with the donor in the future (if they so desire). The level of closeness with the donor is first defined by the parents and the donor (and then when more mature, the child). Closeness may shift and change as these relationships develop over time. It is possible for a child to grow up knowing their donor and other children conceived from the same donor (i.e. so-called donor siblings), and contact and a sense of closeness to a varying degree. These relationships can evolve and be facilitated through clinics (with appropriate legal considerations), national (e.g. UK Donor Conceived Register and Donor Sibling Link, both HFEA), international donor registers and family efforts facilitated by social media and online websites (e.g. genetic ancestry). Research to date suggests that some children do try to contact donors out of curiosity or for medical reasons [20]. Only in rare situations do such contacts result in difficulties but too little research exists to draw firm conclusions. Future studies tracing how the 2005 law impacts on family relationships will be needed post 2023 when the first offspring child benefiting from the law will be 18 years old. Donors of children conceived earlier than 2005 have also come forward to re-register as identifiable donors.

11.3.2.3 Support Needs After Treatment and Beyond

Patients who are successful in achieving their parenthood goals with third-party reproduction show parenting and child development that is similar to those not using third-party reproduction. Nevertheless, parents may have support needs as the children develop and mature relating to the use of third-party reproduction, especially relating to disclosing the nature of the child's conception.

Parents and donors often want to know (in advance of treatment) who will know what information about the donor. Some information could be provided at the start of treatment, but its use is likely to be happen later in the child's development. The HFEA tightly regulates the information flow between the intended parent(s), child and donor(s). The HFEA Code of Practice first and foremost caters to the perceived needs of the person conceived with donated gametes. This means that only this person can seek identifying information about the donor. Parents can receive information about the donor but the law treats such information exchange as meaningful only because it perceives that it will be used to benefit the child and their identity story rather than to satisfy the personal needs of the parent per se. Fertility care staff should become familiar with the information clinics must provide (Table 11.3).

The HFEA recommends that patients be given information about suitable resources to help them with disclosure such as the names of family support groups (i.e. Donor Conception Network) or specialised books (e.g. 'Telling & Talking' series from Donor Conception Network). In general, the recommendation is that children should be told early (between the ages of 3 and 6 years; see [4]) so they have a sense that they have always known, making it more likely this fact is integrated into their self-identity. Disclosure to children needs to be age-appropriate and change as the child matures. There are some challenges to disclosure (see Box 11.3). If parents opt not to disclose to their child then implications of this decision and its accordance with parental values (e.g. openness and honesty) should be discussed. It is likely that patients will in due course want to discuss with an infertility counsellor how and when to talk with their child(ren) about their genetic origins as the child develops. Such discussions often result in further issues to be explored in counselling. For example, teenagers and young adults may express a need to know the donor but their parent(s) may be uncertain about how to meet that need or feel this need threatens their parental role.

It is of key importance that clinicians also consider the needs for support among those patients whose treatment was not successful, and whose desire to become parents in this way was frustrated. The Code of Practice states that counselling be offered before, during and after treatment. In a systematic review of evidence published between 1978 and 2015, there was compelling evidence that psychosocial care directed at

Table 11.3 Information UK clinics have to provide to parents, donor and offspring on request child according to law

Donor conceived persons	Recipient parent(s)	Donors
• At 16 years of age: non-identifying information about the donor (e.g. religion, occupation) and donor sibling(s) (e.g. number of siblings, their gender, medical history). • At 18 years of age: name and last known address of donor and contact with any genetic donor sibling(s) who are registered on HFEA Donor Sibling Link and willing to have contact. • Offer of psychosocial counselling is mandatory before being provided with identifying information about the donor. The HFEA offers a free counselling and intermediary service.	• Non-identifying information (e.g. religion, occupation, phenotype) about the donor(s) whose gametes will or have been used in their treatment. • Can also apply to the HFEA to access basic information about the number, year of birth and sex of any donor sibling(s) up until their donor-conceived child is 18 years of age.	• Donors have a statutory right to request and be provided with basic information of the number of offspring born from their donation, their years of birth and their sex.

See ref. [25].

Box 11.3 Challenges in Disclosing to the Child That They Were Conceived with Donated Gametes

Disclosure needs to be revisited repeatedly because children's understanding develops as they develop and mature.

Young children may [inadvertently] tell others, for example, friends, teachers or even strangers.

Grandparents may be supportive but research shows some may also disregard the fact and its implications, or be ambivalent or even hostile to it.

Disclosure must be made in a way that is congruent with existing family relationships.

Some families and children using third-party reproduction may be stigmatised; ethnicity and race is likely to matter, as is sexuality and family form.

Some families may keep use of donated gametes secret to safeguard vital intergenerational relationships and support for themselves and their children.

Informing others necessarily reveals the infertility problems (if applicable).

Parents may worry that disclosure will negatively affect family dynamics, that the child will be drawn towards the donor or that the child will develop a relationship with the donor.

See refs. [2, 4, 5].

---

helping women and couples relinquish their parenting goals was needed in all forms of fertility care. The review add reference recommended that psychosocial support should target meaning-making processes, acceptance and the pursuit of new life goals to aid longer term psychosocial adjustment (see MyJourney, their support program: https://myjourney.pt).

11.3.2.4 Assessing the Suitability of Intended Parents, Donors and Surrogates

The law requires that any treatment services regulated by the HFEA be provided only after account has been taken of the welfare of any child born as a result of the treatment and of any other child that might be affected by that birth. This is a very important component of assessment prior to treatment (for in-depth details see Section 8, HFEA Code of Practice [1]). This is to be carried out with each intended parent(s) (and their partner if they have one) and without prejudice (on grounds of protected characteristics e.g. race, disability, sexual orientation). In the case of surrogacy, the assessment applies to the intended parent(s) as well as the surrogate and her partner (if there is one), due to the possibility that the surrogate could decide to parent the child. Gamete and embryo donors and people storing gametes for future use do not have to be assessed, as they will not be parents or not intending to be parents now. The exception to this are those donating as part of their own infertility treatment process (i.e., egg and sperm shares). Diverse factors should be considered (Box 11.4). If patients are refused treatment then they should be fully informed in writing of why that decision was made, given the opportunity to

---

Box 11.4 Factors to Consider for Welfare of the Child Assessment

Factors to consider for welfare of the child assessment are past or present patient or partner circumstances (where relevant) likely to cause to any child who may be born or to any existing child of the family serious physical or psychological harm or neglect or lack of care (or of supportive parenting) throughout childhood:

- Previous convictions relating to harming children
- Child protection measures taken regarding existing children
- Violence or serious discord in the family environment
- Mental or physical conditions
- Drug or alcohol abuse
- Medical history, where the medical history indicates that any child who may be born is likely to suffer from a serious medical condition
- Circumstances that the center considers likely to cause serious harm to any aforementioned child

Note. 'Supportive parenting is a commitment to the health, wellbeing and development of the child. It is presumed that all prospective parents will be supportive parents, in the absence of any reasonable cause for concern that any child who may be born, or any other child, may be at risk of significant harm or neglect. Where centers have a concern as to whether this commitment exists, they may wish to take account of wider family and social networks within which the child will be raised.' (HFEA Code of Practice, Section 8.14).

---

provide additional information and to receive appropriate counselling to be able to overcome any challenges to the use of third-party reproduction. In the case of surrogacy, the HFEA expects the 'treating clinician' (Section 8, HFEA Code of Practice) to make the decision about the welfare of the child and document the evidence used to make it. However, it does not make clear who should make welfare of the child decisions for other types of treatment.

11.3.2.5 Implication Discussion and Psychosocial Counselling for Donors, Surrogates and Their Partners

The HFEA requirement to prepare people for treatment includes preparation for the donor, surrogate and their partners. They too need to fully understand the arrangement and its long-term implications for them and be offered suitable opportunities for infertility counselling. There are many practical and medical aspects of how the treatment will be delivered and this information should be provided in as much detail as is needed for informed consent (e.g. procedure, time investment, screening and implications of screening, financial compensation, legislation, recording and potential use of personal data). All parties to third-party donation and surrogacy should be informed that direct-to-consumer DNA testing makes it possible for any of them to be traced if their DNA, or that of a relative, is added to a database holding such information (e.g. ancestry, donor registries).

In addition, clinicians should become familiar with the general psychosocial implications for all donors (egg, sperm, embryo, mitochondrial), surrogates and partners of donors and surrogates (Table 11.4) and acquire more in-depth knowledge about the specific groups they work with (see HFEA Code of Practice for requirements of different treatment groups). For example, women who become egg donors in exchange for reduced treatment costs ('egg sharing') must be informed of the number of eggs to be donated and which woman will receive the additional egg if an odd number of eggs is retrieved. Also important, is for the egg donor to consider that the recipient of their donation may become pregnant but they may not. These are not issues that people donating gametes outside a benefit in kind arrangement will face. Newer forms of donation (e.g. mitochondrial) require particular care pathways for which outcomes are not yet known (e.g. neurodevelopment in children) and for which specialised care pathways, staff and counsellors are required.

In all cases, the HFEA recommends that donors, surrogates and their partners should have the opportunity to have a discussion about implications with a specialised infertility counsellor because it is likely that such discussions could raise emotional and psychological issues. If the donor elects not to have infertility counselling then such a discussion should take place with a member of the staff with sufficient skill, experience and knowledge of these treatments and of patients undergoing these treatments to have a thorough discussion of the implications of treatment.

Table 11.4 Implications to be discussed with donors and surrogates (and their partners, if applicable)

Donors (sperm, egg, embryos), surrogates and their partners

In-depth exploration of motives to ensure an independent and voluntary decision (especially in intra-familial arrangements)

Reflection on what it means now, and potentially in the future, to have a child conceived with their gametes, embryo or their surrogacy, living in a different family; these perceptions may change over time (e.g. after becoming a mother, father, when in a new relationship, or in the case of future infertility and so on)

Their wishes about the desired relationship with the future family of intended parent(s) and their own family (i.e. the donor child will be a half-sibling to their children, if any)

Level of support desired from their partner and wider family and networks (especially surrogate)

The requirement for their screening and implications of unexpected adverse discovery

Become knowledgeable about current possibilities of tracing via DNA testing

Surrogates (additional to above)

The surrogate (and partner) will be assessed to take account of the welfare of the potential child born from treatment and any other child affected by the use of treatment. Donors do not have to be assessed.

There could be a breakdown in the surrogacy arrangement; the surrogate may not wish to relinquish the baby or sign the parental order. All parties should draw up a surrogacy agreement and be comfortable with its content. The UK government provides detailed guidance on surrogacy arrangements.

Embryo donation

A young person conceived at the same time and genetically related to their own children (i.e. full sibling) may contact them in the future.

Mitochondrial donation

Meaning for the family of nuclear versus mitochondrial DNA (e.g. views on three parent families)

See refs. [2–5].

11.4 Global Perspectives on Third-Party Reproduction

This section explores two additional key issues to be considered in the context of patients' psychosocial experiences and implication discussions: the growing number of patients travelling to and from the United Kingdom to access desired reproductive services and the technologies that impact on the nature and use of reproductive technologies worldwide.

11.4.1 Cross Border Reproductive Services

In 2010, based on a survey of 46 clinics in six European countries, it was estimated that 11,000 to 14,000 patients were travelling to and from diverse European countries to receive reproductive services. This type of care is referred to as cross border reproductive services (CBRS). CBRS produces a rich diversity in the populations fertility care staff are likely to encounter in their clinics. Doctors should understand the context of CBRS and be prepared to manage patients travelling to or from abroad for services.

Reasons for Using Cross Border Reproductive Care

People undertake CBRC for many reasons, for example, prohibition of treatment option, lack of donors, long waiting lists, high costs and non-anonymous or anonymous third-party reproduction being prohibited in home country. To illustrate, there are couples from Germany and Switzerland who have chosen the United Kingdom for egg donation, as they consider it vital for their children to be able to access the identity of the donor in the future (P. Thorn, personal communication, 31 January 2019). Conversely, UK couples travel to the United States for surrogacy because they perceive legal processes to be easier. It is vital that clinicians are aware of the variations in laws on third-party reproduction in different countries and the kinds of challenges patients might face in going abroad or coming to the United Kingdom from abroad (Box 11.5). Surrogacy illustrates the variations in national laws and the pace of change worldwide. Access to surrogacy in a European context is very limited (e.g. illegal in France, Germany, Austria, Switzerland, Norway and Sweden). India and Thailand were significant providers of surrogacy for European heterosexual and same-sex male couples, but both countries have recently limited access as a result of cross country cases with dubious outcomes (see 'Japanese baby gets birth certificate', *The Hindu*, 11 August, 2008, ('Japanese baby gets birth certificate'). India barred access for gay couples in 2012, and commercial surrogacy altogether in 2017. Thailand barred access for foreign couples in 2015.

> **Box 11.5** Types of Legal and Practice Variations in National Policies on Cross Border Reproductive Services
>
> - Accessibility of some treatments (e.g. surrogacy)
> - Legality of gamete donation (egg, sperm and embryo donation) and surrogacy
> - Availability of donors
> - Treatment costs
> - Perceived success rates
> - Perceived legal ease
> - Age requirements of the treatment seeker
> - Accessibility for LGBT communities

The USA remains a major destination for surrogacy, and emerging destinations for gay and heterosexual surrogacy include, for example, Mexico.

11.4.2 Challenges of Cross Border Reproductive Services for Patients Seeking Third-Party Reproduction in the United Kingdom or Abroad

Delivery of treatment services in the United Kingdom for patients from abroad (incoming) follow the same standards and code of practice as care delivered to patients from the United Kingdom (e.g. information provision, implication discussion, offer of counselling). UK citizens having treatment abroad (outgoing) will be covered by legislation (if it exists) in the country providing treatment. It is possible that clinics in the United Kingdom and abroad have made arrangements for comparability of treatment. Also, donors and surrogates should be informed and consent to donating to intended parents from abroad. CBRS poses some practical challenges to clinics (e.g. language barriers, access to historical notes, follow-up care, different expectations of care), and these challenges can be experienced as stressful for staff and patients. CBRS poses particular challenges to intended parents, as many are unaware of the legal and policy framework of treatment abroad and are unknowledgeable about the medical system. There seems to be a lack of accessible and reliable information for CBRS, and many patients base their choices on online-information provided by clinics abroad (incoming, outgoing). This poverty of information is particularly pertinent for patients travelling to access treatment prohibited in their home country, since information could also be banned. Therefore, people using CBRS (incoming or outgoing) could be a vulnerable group, and clinic staff ensuring discussions about implications and access to infertility (psychosocial) counselling is essential (see Table 11.5). Implications counselling for incoming patients should be provided by clinics (as required by law). These patients should have access to an interpreter or advocate (if needed), and in keeping with best practice, family members should not be used as interpreters. Outgoing patients are unlikely to be under a UK clinic's duty of care and consequently will most likely need to arrange implications counselling privately.

Internet and Medical Developments Impacting Third-Party Reproduction

The Internet and new medical technologies are an increasingly important dimension to consider in the context of third-party reproduction, shaping the psychosocial landscape of intended parents, donors and donor conceived offspring.

We cannot under-estimate the importance of the Internet as a major source to which people go to learn about the process of third-party reproduction, for example, to find out information about clinics, their success rates, accessibility of different forms of third-party reproduction, surrogacy, pricing and access issues in the United Kingdom and abroad. The social networking capacity (e.g. Facebook, online donor registries) of the Internet has, in recent years, given rise to informal approaches to third-party reproduction (see Box 11.6). Fertility staff need to be aware of the possibilities that recipients and donors may move between the informal online world and the more formal clinical world as they pursue parenthood goals. Fertility care staff should be prepared to discuss the opportunities and risks of these informal practices.

Also on the horizon are important developments of new reproductive technologies and techniques, for example, genome editing, human cloning, the development of artificial wombs and gametes, parthenogenesis and so on. These are raising a series of new and important questions for third-party reproduction, which will no doubt impact on patient populations and implications discussions in the future.

11.5 Conclusions

Counselling in third-party reproduction is complex and requires knowledge in the practical and medical

Table 11.5 Additional counselling issues prior to cross border treatment according to group

Intended parents	Donors/surrogates	Offspring
• Explore motivation and expectation of treatment abroad. • Raise awareness of potential language barriers, cultural differences; provide information about counselling in the native language of patients (e.g. infertility counselling organisations in home country). • Explore financial, emotional, psychological and other resources required to carry out treatment abroad. • Understand costs, compensation for donors/surrogates as well as typical treatment for donor/surrogate to judge whether these are reasonable (or appropriate) and ethical. • Inform about legal regulation of treatment planned in country of treatment, esp. regarding access to information about donor/legal parentage after surrogacy. • If intended parents plan treatment prohibited in their home country, they need to consider the implications for themselves and intended children (i.e. manage shame, insecurity, disclosure).	• Prior asking for consent to accepting intended parents from abroad; clinic may not be able to inform about pregnancy and birth abroad. • Explore situation where offspring from abroad wishes contact with donor; implications for donor and their family (biological relatives across countries). • Manage language barrier between donor/surrogate (and their family) and offspring. • Explore emotional dimensions of exported gametes, if applicable.	• Make offspring aware of potential complexity involved in seeking donor/surrogate if some form of CBRC has taken place (i.e. offspring lives in country with access to donor, but treatment was in country with anonymity). • Manage biological relatives, potentially across several countries. • Manage language barrier between donor/surrogate (and their family) and offspring.

Box 11.6 Effects of the Internet on Informal Practice of Third-Party Reproduction

- To find donors or intended co-parents (especially lesbians and single women).
- Networking and contact among donor conceived offspring, parents and donors, for example, via the genetic databases or online platforms such as the Donor Sibling Registry (at any age) or the HFEA registry (at age 18 years).
- (Young) people may use direct-to-consumer genetic testing kits to find biological relatives. These have become more affordable and available to the general population.
- Donors and donor conceived people may be traced if their DNA, or that of a relative, is added to a database, making donor anonymity more difficult for past and present donors.

See refs. [2, 4].

---

aspects of treatment but also in psychosocial and legal areas. The HFEA Code of Practice makes clear that all parties to any arrangement using third-party reproduction should be counselled (intended parents, donors, surrogates and their partners, any existing children). Counselling (psychosocial and for discussion of implications) should be offered and available throughout the treatment process and later stages for families involved (offspring thus conceived, any other offspring affected and family as well as donor/surrogate and family).

Staff with experience, knowledge and skills in the specified treatment can provide discussions of implications of using third-party reproduction. However, the HFEA recommends that such discussions be provided by specialised infertility counsellors trained to also assist with psychosocial aspects of third-party reproduction. It is important that healthcare professionals providing patient support and counselling be aware of the complexity of the issues involved for patients (including relational, social, financial and legal ones) and also of the variation of experience in different patient groups.

Supporting patients in third-party reproduction is best achieved through close collaboration between all members of staff involved in providing care to ensure consistent information and counselling content for donors, surrogates, their partners and intended parents and children.

Assisted reproductive technology is a highly dynamic field and there are many new developments on the horizon, requiring regular updating of knowledge. For example, the use of cross border reproductive services and mitochondrial donations is increasing but studies are still underway to fully understand the implications of these forms of third-party reproduction. New technologies such as gene editing could further impact on third-party reproduction. Finally, the way third-party reproduction is arranged and family situations created and developed over time are increasingly shaped by social media and online platforms. Fertility clinics and staff need to keep pace with these developments to support patients wanting to be involved in third-party reproduction.

References

1. Human Fertilisation and Embryology Authority. Code of Practice. 9th ed., London; 2019. Available at: www .hfea.gov.uk/media/2609/june-2018-code-of-practice-9th-edition-draft.pdf (accessed 4 February 2019).

2. Committee on Quality of Healthcare in America, Institute of Medicine. *Improving the 21st century healthcare system: crossing the quality chasm. A new health system for the 21st century.* Washington, DC: National Academies Press; 2001, 39–60.

3. Dancet EA, Nelen WL, Sermeus W, De Leeuw L, Kremer JA, D'Hooghe TM. The patients' perspective on fertility care: a systematic review. *Hum Reprod Update.* 2010;**16**(5):467–87.

4. Dancet EAF, Van Empel IWH, Rober P, Nelen WLDM, Kremer JAM, d'Hooghe TM. Patient-centred infertility care: a qualitative study to listen to the patient's voice. *Hum Reprod.* 2011;**26**(4):827–33.

6. Human Fertilisation and Embryology Authority. *Code of Practice*, 7th ed. London; 2009.

7. Nordqvist P, Smart C. *Relative strangers: family life, genes and donor conception.* London: Palgrave Macmillan; 2014.

8. Human Fertilisation and Embryology Authority. Fertility treatment 2014–2016: trends and figures. 2018. Available at: www.hfea.gov.uk/media/2563/hfea-fertility-trends-and-figures-2017-v2.pdf (accessed 31 January 2019).

9. Graham S. Being a 'good' parent: single women reflecting upon 'selfishness' and 'risk' when pursuing motherhood through sperm donation. *Anthropol Med.* 2017;**25**(3):249–64.

10. Jadva V, Badger S, Morrissette M, Golombok S. 'Mom by choice, single by life's circumstance . . . ': Findings from a large scale survey of the experiences of single mothers by choice. *Hum Fertil.* 2009;**12**(4):175–84.

11. Nordqvist P. 'Out of sight, out of mind': family resemblances in lesbian donor conception. *Sociology.* 2010;**44**(6):1128–44.

13. Quiroga S. Blood is thicker than water: policing donor insemination and the reproduction of whiteness. *Hypatia.* 2007;**22**(2):143–61.

14. Ariza L. Keeping up appearances in the Argentine fertility clinic: making kinship visible through race in donor conception. *Tecnoscienza.* 2015;**6**(1):5–31.

15. Andreassen R. *Mediated kinship: gender, race and sexuality in donor families.* London: Routledge;2019.

16. Nordqvist P. Dealing with sperm: comparing lesbians' clinical and non-clinical donor conception processes. *Sociol Health Illness.* 2011;**33**(1):114–29.

17. Donovan C, Heaphy B, Weeks J. *Same sex intimacies: families of choice and other life experiments.* New York: Routledge;2001.

18. Freeman T, Jadva V, Tranfield E, Golombok S. Online sperm donation: a survey of the demographic characteristics, motivations, preferences and experiences of sperm donors on a connection website. *Hum Reprod.* 2016;**31**(9):2082–9.

19. Jadva V, Freeman T, Tranfield E., Golombok S. 'Friendly allies in raising children': a survey of men and women seeking elective co-parenting arrangements via an online connection website. *Hum Reprod.* 2015;**30** (8):1896–906.

20. Jadva V, Freeman T, Kramer W, Golombok S. Sperm and oocyte donors' experiences of anonymous donation and subsequent contact with their donor offspring. *Hum Reprod.* 2010;638–45.

22. Shelton KH, Boivin J, Hay D, et al. Examining differences in psychological adjustment problems among children conceived by assisted reproductive technologies. *IntJ Behav Dev.* 2009;**33**(5):385–92.

25. Gilman L, Nordqvist P. Organising openness: how UK policy defines the significance of information and information sharing about gamete donation. *Int J Law Policy Family.* 2018;**32**(3):316–33.

26. Montuschi O. Telling and talking series. The Donor Conception Network. 2019. Available at: www .dcnetwork.org/catalog/telling-and-talking-series (accessed 31 January 2019).

27. Thorn P, Wischmann T. German guidelines for psychosocial counselling in the area of gamete donation. *Hum Fertil.* 2009;**12**(2):73–80.

28. Culley L, Hudson N. Public understandings of science: British South Asian men's perception of third party assisted conception. *Int J Interdisciplin Soc Sci.* 2007;**2** (4):79–86.

30. Gameiro S, Finnigan A. Long-term adjustment to unmet parenthood goals following ART: a systematic review and meta-analysis. *Hum Reprod Update.* 2017;**3** (1):322–37.

31. Gorman GS, McFarland R, Stewart J, Feeney C, Turnbull DM. Mitochondrial donation: from test tube to clinic. *Lancet.* 2018;**392**(10154): 1191–2.

32. Dimond R. Social and ethical issues in mitochondrial donation. *British Med Bull.* 2015;**115**(1):173.

33. Shenfield F, De Mouzon J, Pennings G, et al. ESHRE Taskforce on Cross Border Reproductive Care. Cross border reproductive care in six European countries. *Hum Reprod.* 2010;**25**(6):1361–8.

35. Salama M, Isachenko V, Isachenko E, et al. Cross border reproductive care (CBRC): a growing global phenomenon with multidimensional implications (a systematic and critical review). *J Assist Reprod Genet.* 2018;1–12.

36. Japanese baby gets birth certificate. *The Hindu*, 11 August 2008. Available at www.thehindu.com/todays-paper/tp-national/tp-otherstates/Japanese-baby-gets-birth-certificate/article15278695.ece (accessed 4 February 2019).

37. Blyth E, Thorn P, Wischmann T. CBRC and psychosocial counselling: assessing needs and developing an ethical framework for practice. *Reprod Biomed Online.* 2011;**23**(5):642–51.

38. Culley L, Hudson N, Rapport F, Blyth E, Norton W, Pacey AA. Crossing borders for fertility treatment: motivations, destinations and outcomes of UK fertility travellers. *Hum Reprod.* 2011;**26**(9):2373–81.

39. Boivin J, Bunting L, Koert E, ieng UC, Verhaak C. Perceived challenges of working in a fertility clinic: a qualitative analysis of work stressors and difficulties working with patients. *Hum Reprod.* 2017;**32**(2):403–8.

40. Thorn P, Wischmann T, Blyth E. Cross-border reproductive services–suggestions for ethically based minimum standards of care in Europe. *J Psychosom Obstet Gynecol.* 2012;**33**(1):1–6.

41. Thorn P. Cross border medically assisted reproduction from a psychosocial perspective-legal challenges and the welfare of the child. *Cult Res.* 2016;**5**:317–30.

42. Harper J, Kennett D, Reisel D. The end of donor anonymity: how genetic testing is likely to drive anonymous gamete donation out of business. *Hum Reprod.* 2016;**31**(6):1135–40.

43. Greely HT. *The end of sex and the future of human reproduction.* Cambridge, MA: Harvard University Press; 2016.

44. Romanis EC. Artificial womb technology and the frontiers of human reproduction: conceptual differences and potential implications. *J Med Ethics.* 2018;**44**:751–5.

Further Reading

Crawshaw MK, Daniels D, Adam K, et al. Emerging international models for facilitating contact between people genetically related through donor conception and their implications for donor conception fertility treatment services. *Reprod Biomed Soc Online.* 2015;**1** (2):71–80.

Gameiro S, Boivin J, Dancet E, et al. ESHRE guideline: routine psychosocial care in infertility and medically assisted reproduction—a guide for fertility staff. *Hum Reprod.* 2015;**30**(11):2476–85.

Golombok S. *Modern families: parents and children in new family forms.* Cambridge: Cambridge University Press; 2015.

Hudson N, Culley L, Blyth E, Norton W, Rapport F, Pacey A. 2011. Cross-border reproductive care: a review of the literature. *Reprod Biomed Online.* **22** (7):673–85.

Nordqvist P. The drive for openness in donor conception: disclosure and the trouble with real life. *Int J Law Policy Family.* 2014;**28**(3):321–38.

Söderström-Anttila, V., Wennerholm, U.B., Loft, A., et al. Surrogacy: outcomes for surrogate mothers, children and the resulting families – a systematic review. *Hum Reprod Update.* 2015;**22**(2): 260–76.

Chapter 12

Managing Ethical Dilemmas in Reproductive Medicine

Gillian Lockwood

12.1 Introduction

From our current standpoint, it is difficult to imagine that more than 40 years ago, the birth of Louise Brown, the pioneering achievement of Steptoe and Edwards, was hailed not just with admiration and joy but also with hostility. Critics pointed to the 'low' success rates (105 embryo transfers before a healthy birth), and many commented on the high cost (which would inevitably limit access to the wealthy few in the richer countries). Some religious authorities forbade its use for their adherents, claiming that it was 'unnatural' and morally repugnant. Some social commentators considered it to mark another potential slip down the 'slope' that could lead to the commodification and commercialisation of human reproduction.

Clinicians and scientists working in the field of fertility are still confronted by opposition and misunderstanding, and the media frequently misrepresent what has been achieved or may be possible in the future. It is therefore vital that we have a solid grasp of the ethical basis of our work and can explain and justify what we do with conviction. In no other branch of medicine is 'Primum non nocere (above all, do no harm)' so central.

Since Beauchamp and Childress published their seminal book on biomedical ethics in 2001, it has become almost conventional wisdom to analyse medical ethical problems and dilemmas in terms of their 'Four Principles': Autonomy, Beneficence (the promotion of good), the avoidance of harm (nonmaleficence) and Justice. Patient autonomy is considered to be the most important that effectively trumps the other three (Figure 12.1).

This may seem a welcome inversion after centuries of medical 'paternalism' meant that patients didn't expect to question their doctor's decisions about their care or even to understand the nature of their diagnosis and prognosis. However, given the special circumstances of modern reproductive medicine, it is important to examine how far such 'principlism' should be applied to the management of ethical dilemmas in assisted reproductive technology (ART).

The potential for modern fertility treatment to offer the chance of biological parenthood to otherwise infertile couples, in an environment where patients have expectations of achieving all their goals, inevitably raises questions about both the entitlement to treatment and the nature of that provision.

12.2 Why Is Fertility Medicine Different?

Fertility treatment differs from other branches of medicine in two fundamental respects. First, the fertility patient is not 'ill' in any conventional sense even though their infertility may have a pathological basis. Infertility may be a source of significant morbidity causing depression and social dysfunction, but most people, and even most clinicians, would regard infertility more as a disadvantage or handicap such as extreme myopia or low intelligence. However, in some cultures, childlessness (which is still seen as a predominantly female 'problem') is a huge social stigma and the failure to 'produce' a child may result in divorce or extreme neglect. Second, infertility treatment is perceived as being generally 'unsuccessful' and is compared unfavourably with other treatments of acute conditions in surgery or therapeutics. This widespread perception is clearly mistaken, as modern fertility treatments offer cumulative success rates over several cycles of treatment that compare favourably with those of a normally fertile couple trying to conceive naturally.

Even in cases in which extraordinary procedures are required such as ovum donation for premature ovarian failure (POF) or percutaneous epididymal sperm aspiration (PESA) with intracytoplasmic sperm injection (ICSI) for obstructive azoospermia

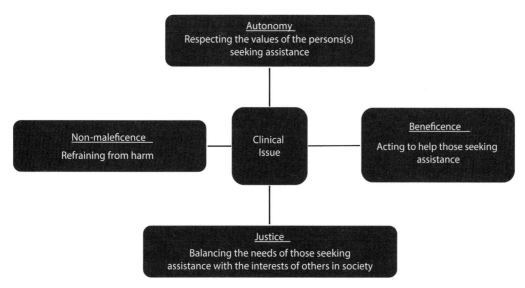

Figure 12.1 Ethical principles in reproductive medicine.
Source: After Beauchamp T, Childress J. *Principles of biomedical ethics*, 4th ed. New York: Oxford University Press, 1994.

the eventual outcome of treatment is likely to be influenced more by lack of resources to provide the treatments required than by deficiencies in the techniques available.

Philosophical purists often claim that the successful delivery of a baby is not a 'cure' for infertility because the couple remain infertile as long as they rely on technology to assist them to procreate. This is sheer sophistry; a baby is a cure of infertility in exactly the same way as a beta blocker is a cure for hypertension. There may be some psychological benefits for the ultimately unsuccessful couple in just undertaking fertility treatment in that they may feel that at least their needs have been recognised and they have taken the opportunity to challenge their fate. However, one significant disadvantage of fertility treatment is that the desired outcome, the safe delivery of a healthy baby, is an 'all or nothing' event. Unsuccessful treatment can rarely offer palliation or therapeutic benefit in the way that a less than wholly successful operation may offer an acceptable if suboptimal outcome. Indeed a 'biochemical' pregnancy or early miscarriage following treatment may be perceived as 'worse' than a negative test.

Long-term follow-up studies of couples who embarked on fertility treatment but were ultimately unable to achieve a successful pregnancy have shown that they do suffer significantly initially in terms of depression and regret, but that over time (five to seven years) they return to levels of life satisfaction that compare favourably with the levels of those who did succeed with fertility treatment and with the spontaneously fertile. As would be expected, individuals who make a 'positive' decision to abandon further fertility treatment after repeated failures fare better than those who wished to continue but could not undertake further treatment because of age or resource allocation.

In clinical terms, the decision to offer fertility treatment has significantly different implications from all other (successful) clinical interventions. In treating other medical problems, successful end results clearly affect the patients, their relatives and to some extent the wider society, but a successful fertility treatment involves an additional party in the child who is born. This individual's very existence inevitably has a significant influence on all other social and family relationships; indeed the arrival of the child may create the family.

12.3 Considering Possible People

To what extent the clinician needs to consider the potential existence of this, as yet un-conceived child, is a complex philosophical issue. The interests of people who may be born as a result of fertility treatment clearly are not as tangible as those of existing people, but legislation governing the application of the new reproductive technologies sets great store by the interests of the (possible) child. The Human

Fertilisation and Embryology Act (1991) states that 'centres considering treatment must take into account the welfare of any child that may be born'. From that standpoint it would seem difficult to justify restricting availability or access to treatments except in the limiting case where the expected quality of life of the child is so low that the child might realistically wish that he or she had never been born. All other children born as a result of fertility treatment (1.5% of all babies born in the United Kingdom and 8 million worldwide since 1987 following in vitro fertilisation [IVF]) represent a significant addition to the sum of human happiness, and this is so even if we ignore the happiness of their parents and relations.

It may seem that adding the interests of the 'potential person' to an equation for setting medical priorities in therapies that include fertility treatment involves a significant problem of incommensurability: how do we weigh the interests of 'potential' against those of 'actual' people? £5000 could 'buy' an IVF cycle for a young couple who, with fresh and subsequent, frozen embryo transfers, could realistically achieve the birth of at least one healthy child. That same £5000 would make very little contribution to the cost of providing 'reprogrammed' chimeric antigen receptor T cell (CAR T) therapy for a child with leukaemia who had relapsed after conventional treatment and which is currently estimated at £300,000.

The inevitable conclusion must be that withholding fertility treatment on the grounds of the interest of the 'welfare of the child' is a philosophically unsustainable position. Whether this is equivalent to claiming that we have a positive duty to 'make more' happy people is equally contentious. Perhaps this is a political rather than an ethical decision. Many governments have promoted pro-natalist policies because of concern about declining populations and falling birth rates, and in the era of ART, some governments are actively supporting state-funded fertility treatment as a way of ensuring that their citizens (usually the educated, professional classes who are most likely to be childless) are encouraged and helped to have children.

12.4 Ethical Approaches

12.4.1 Consequentialism

Conventional medical ethics theory tends to be divided into consequentialist doctrines that purport to evaluate the outcome of clinical decisions in terms of consequences, good or bad, and rights- or rule-based systems that judge clinical decisions and outcomes in terms of the extent to which a 'right' is advanced or a 'good' rule applied. In the simplest case, a single successful cycle of IVF for a childless couple resulting in the birth of a healthy baby seems to be a purely positive outcome. On the basis of a cost–benefit analysis, the financial costs are modest (even allowing for the opportunity cost of diverting scarce resources to fertility treatment) and the foreseeable medium- and long-term consequences are equally positive.

Some potential negative consequences may be foreseen. For example, the child may be neglected or abused, or the couple's relationship may founder under the psychological stress of even a successful cycle, but these are rare cases. As a society we recognise that a significant proportion of births are unplanned and accidental (50% according to some surveys), yet we would be horrified at the prospect of spontaneously fertile people being required to fulfil the criteria of 'suitability to parent' that some treatment centres impose on their patients in the name of equity or the 'interests of the child'. One in five babies born in the United Kingdom grow up in a household with no father, but single women seeking to become mothers in a safe and lawful way face significant obstacles in accessing treatment and the financial burden is high.

12.4.2 Comparisons with Adoption

Consider the analogy that is often drawn between allocating access to fertility treatment and authorities 'choosing' the best possible adoptive parents for a baby who has been given up at birth by its mother. Given the 'shortage' of healthy newborns available for adoption in the United Kingdom, and the large number of couples who would like to adopt a baby, it is generally accepted that the authorities must 'choose' the 'best' possible would-be parents for that child. But given the large number of children taken into our care homes, whose life outcomes are recognised to be very compromised, do we, as a society, accept that possibly 'lower' standards of potential parenting may be acceptable for prospective adoptive parents in these cases? Caring though half-competent parenting is infinitely preferable for 'looked after' children who have been rescued from neglect and abuse to them remaining in Institutions.

This is clearly a false analogy to make with decisions about the provision of fertility treatment. The child who may, or even will, be born as the result of successful fertility treatment can be born only to the would-be parents who came to the fertility clinic. They may not be, potentially, the 'best' parents, but they are the only parents that this, as yet unconceived, child can have.

12.4.3 Rights-Based Systems of Ethics

Rights-based systems are ethically more contentious. Article 12 of the European Convention on Human Rights does protect the right to 'found a family', but this legislation was drawn up at a time when an individual's right not to be compulsorily sterilised was the issue at stake, and in the era before ART was even envisaged. There can be no right to have a child, in the sense that somebody, possibly society, has a corresponding duty to provide successful fertility treatment. Demand for medical treatment, including fertility treatment, is theoretically unlimited because even in wealthy countries there will always be a disparity between what individuals could theoretically benefit from and what society can afford to provide. For this reason, the concept of rationing in healthcare, including fertility treatment, is accepted and the issue becomes one of ensuring justice, equity of distribution or simply rationing 'fairly'.

12.4.5 Fairness

'Justice as Fairness' requires a balancing of needs and deserts. In an acute or progressive clinical situation, the condition itself generates its own therapeutic agenda. Responsible clinicians treat the life-threatening and rapidly deteriorating conditions before the mild and stable, and little or no consideration is given either to the cost of the intervention, the responsibility of the patients for their condition or even the likelihood of a successful outcome. A computer algorithm that could predict the outcome of admission of a patient to an ITU with 98% accuracy (and therefore save the pain, anguish and expense of often a prolonged and ultimately futile time spent in intensive care) was condemned as inhumane. Yet, decisions about access to funded (or even private) fertility treatment are made on criteria with much less statistical rigour such as anti-mullerian hormone (AMH) levels or body mass index (BMI).

However, infertility patients are generally not perceived to be in this position, however great their distress. The condition itself does not deteriorate except in the sense that advancing female age may eventually make it less likely to succeed. Funding commissioners may feel entitled to consider the issue of desert and responsibility in the field of infertility treatment when they would not in any other medical arena. Diabetics who smoke or transplant patients who do not comply with their medication will still be treated, unlike fertility patients who are often held to be 'responsible' for their childlessness. Patients report, through tears, of being asked, 'Why didn't you start trying for a baby when you were younger?' or 'How do you think you got the Chlamydia that has blocked your tubes?'! Even when the needs of all infertile people are recognised, allocation of resources is often made on the basis of personal desert or utility. A 30-year-old childless married woman with tubal blockage due to peritonitis will be offered IVF on the NHS whereas a 36-year-old, previously sterilised, mother of two cannot get the treatment she needs to have a baby with her new partner. When discussing questions of need in this context, the issue is one of how to allocate limited resources so that utility is maximised and injustice is minimised. The sheer complexity of human motivation is such that the calculation of needs and deserts is fraught with difficulty, and that is assuming that we can answer the fundamental question of whether the fertile five-sixths of the population or the decision makers (i.e. the clinicians or commissioners who control access to treatment) are entitled to make judgments about the lifestyles, needs and deserts of the one-sixth of the population who cannot reproduce spontaneously.

Some authorities have claimed that if guidelines for access to fertility treatments can be agreed, then justice demands only that the guidelines are applied impartially: that is, the content of the guidelines is relatively unimportant. This type of 'procedural' justice is exemplified by the 'post-code lottery' that has prevailed in England and Wales notwithstanding the National Institute for Health and Care Excellence (NICE) guideline of 2004 which recommended three 'full' (including frozen embryo transfers) for all eligible childless couples.

A clinician may meet in her NHS fertility clinic, 10 consecutive couples from 10 different Care Commissioning Groups (CCGs), who will all have different criteria for eligibility for treatment (age,

BMI, AMH, time-trying, age of partner, parity, smoking history . . .) and different treatment options (one, two or possibly even three cycles which may include freezing and frozen transfers, may include donor gametes, may even include funded transfer of frozen embryos for a sibling pregnancy).

12.5 The Moral Status of the Human Embryo

The original Human Fertilisation and Embryology Act (1990) and its subsequent iterations accords a special status to human embryos generated in vitro and this has resulted in strict limitations on the nature and extent of embryo research and fertility treatment that can be carried out in the United Kingdom. This special status derives from the embryo's recognised *potential* to become a human being and seems to be in stark contrast to other UK legislation that permits termination of pregnancy at much more advanced gestations than can be currently achieved in vitro.

Notwithstanding different religious perspectives on the point at which 'life' begins (fertilisation, implantation, 'quickening', viability, delivery), it is reasonable to consider at what point in the development of the human organism a creature with a 'right to life' has come into being. If we accept that potential personhood is taken to confer a serious right to life, then the only grounds on which a termination of pregnancy could be defended would be the need to protect the life or health of the mother or the presence in the fetus of an incurable defect that would make its life, if it were to survive, not worth living.

However, we must recognise the political and societal environment in which the field of ART evolved. In 1967, David Steel's Abortion Act permitted termination of pregnancy on a wide number of grounds up to 28 weeks' gestation in Great Britain (but not Northern Ireland). The HFEA Act of 1990 reduced the time limit from 28 to 24 weeks (in the light of developments in neonatal intensive care) and subsequent attempts to reduce the time limit to 22 and 20 weeks have been resisted in Parliament. The implementation of the Steel Act in 1968 occurred just 10 years before Louise Brown's birth and it is clear that attempts to make significant alterations to the HFEA Act risk re-opening the highly politically contentious area of termination of pregnancy.

As the embryologist studies the images of the microscopic cluster of cells which is the blastocyst, they are fully aware that this can progress by an uncertain but inexorable process from the Petri dish to the cradle.

For successful IVF parents too the leap of imagination required to envisage their embryo as a child is very difficult. After successful delivery, however, the supernumerary frozen embryos that represent potential siblings hold a huge, and often painful, emotional significance if the couple do not wish to have further children but feel they cannot donate 'their' children to be brought up by other parents or be allowed to perish. As the 10-year limit on storage draws closer, many couples report that they find the annual letter asking them about their wishes for the disposition of their embryos to be a source of great stress. The default position of paying another year's storage fees seems less than ideal, but many couples rely on the 10-year limit to 'absolve' them of the 'responsibility' of authorising the destruction of their embryos.

12.6 Avoiding the Risks of 'Double Jeopardy' for Fertility Patients with Co-Morbidities

Modern assisted conception can help many individuals achieve genetic parenthood even though they suffer from serious medical problems. Pathologies such as cystic fibrosis were historically associated with short lives and infertility, but now surgical sperm retrieval and ICSI can overcome the azoospermia associated with cystic fibrosis (CF) and men with this condition may prefer genetic fatherhood to using donor sperm. Other serious medical problems may make pregnancy or fatherhood unlikely but not impossible. If an individual with such serious medical problems, for example, if a female post renal transplant patient or a survivor of childhood cancer who required chemotherapy and pelvic irradiation, can achieve a pregnancy naturally, then it is deemed reasonable for the full resources of obstetric and neonatal care to be assembled to support the woman's desire for motherhood. But where assisted conception is required, is it reasonable, given the principle of 'primum non nocere' to try and achieve a pregnancy for someone where there is a non-negligible risk of maternal and/or perinatal death? However, this could be presented as an intolerable example of 'double jeopardy', where an individual who is already unfortunate in their health status is then denied the help they require to achieve a pregnancy. In these circumstances, we have a special duty to balance patient autonomy with the expert opinion of colleagues in cardiology, oncology and transplant medicine who may not share our enthusiasm for IVF!

12.7 Confidentiality and Infertility

Confidentiality is central to the doctor–patient relationship in all branches of medicine, but it is especially so in fertility practice, where patients often feel a sense of shame or guilt about their status. The legislation specifies the care that must be taken not to communicate anything about a patient's fertility care, even that they are having IVF, without their express permission and consent. History taking in fertility consultations is rife with danger and the dual responsibilities of making the right diagnosis by extracting the best history can result in tragedy. There may be emerging secrets: previous unacknowledged paternity, adoption, termination of pregnancy and even sterilisation or gender reassignment may all have an enormous impact on the prospects for treatment outcome and the couple's ongoing relationship.

Fertility doctors rightly stress that infertility is a 'shared' problem and the attribution of 'blame' should be avoided in all but the most obvious cases such as total azoospermia or bilateral tubal blockage. Consultations therefore usually involve both partners simultaneously, but the opportunity should be sought for individual consultations if the history appears inconsistent or implausible.

Extreme sensitivity is required where cultural issues are prominent, for example, in communities where first-cousin marriage has been the norm for multiple generations, the incidence of male subfertility (and fetal anomaly) is quite high. Investigations aimed at identifying a cause of infertility may identify behaviour that can jeopardise a relationship. A man with triple-defect sperm and an abnormal androgen profile finally admitted to five years use of finasteride (bought online) to treat his male pattern hair loss. His wife, who had undergone four failed ICSI cycles, was totally unaware either that he was taking the pills or the effect they were having.

The fertility doctor has a special duty to enhance autonomy by communicating sensitively and effectively so the decision about undertaking fertility treatment and the responsibility for it is shared. It is vital to recognise the limits to accuracy and effectiveness of many diagnostic and therapeutic procedures in fertility practice (and that the patient may have a different perspective).

Some of the basic principles of behavioural economics can assist with managing patient expectations, in that it is vital to recognise that under situations of stress and anxiety people often make apparently 'irrational' decisions and, when faced with complex scenarios, may be incapable of choosing. Fertility treatment is so often expressed in terms of percentages that it is easy to lose sight that percentages apply to populations and not to an individual couple's 'chances' of a baby. Fertility doctors may feel that where female age and ovarian reserve indicate a less than 10% chance of a live birth, then donor eggs are the obvious 'solution'. But for the couple with a 15-year history of primary infertility, even a 10% 'chance' is an option they may wish to consider taking.

12.8 Ethical Dilemmas Arising from the Cryopreservation of Gametes

Since the development in the 1950s of successful sperm cryopreservation it has been possible to separate both temporally and spatially the act of gamete production from that of fertilisation and conception. Technologies of ICSI and surgical sperm retrieval allied with cryopreservation of sperm, oocytes and embryos have revolutionised the way in which society looks at reproductive behaviour and relationships.

Ethical dilemmas can arise from a newfound ability to manipulate our reproductive life span to such an extent that old age and even death are no longer seen as a barrier to having children. It is well recognised that natural fertility and fecundity start to decline quite markedly from the mid-30s in most women with normal reproductive function, and for women in their 40s the chance of achieving a healthy pregnancy, even with IVF, is quite small. The demographic shift that has led women increasingly to defer starting a family until educational, career or financial goals have been achieved has highlighted this mismatch between the life expectancy of women and their reproductive life span. In today's society delayed marriage, divorce and subsequent new relationships are increasingly common.

12.8.1 Posthumous Reproduction and the Cryopreservation of Gametes

Many societies question whether it is acceptable or appropriate for a widow to use frozen embryos that were created with her late husband to give birth to a posthumous child. In the United Kingdom, so long as the correct consent forms have been signed, such treatment is available and the deceased father can have his name put on the baby's birth certificate. In contrast, in France creation of the embryo is viewed as a joint 'project' which ceases to have a purpose on the death of one of the project's originators. In the United States, the uniform anatomical gift act (UAGA), which is in effect in every state gives the next of kin, in designated order of closeness, the right to make material gifts of the deceased's body without limiting the uses that can be made of the gift. Does this authority extend to retrieving gametes to be used by the next of kin for their own reproductive purposes or that of others? Similarly contentious is the use of cryopreserved sperm from a deceased partner to impregnate or otherwise achieve pregnancy in the surviving spouse.

As a society we may wish to consider whether there is any legal or moral distinction in the status of a child who was conceived spontaneously the week before his father's untimely death or that of the child conceived using ART and stored gametes or sperm acquired peri-mortem. Whereas the degree of medical involvement in the three processes is clearly different, nevertheless the child's existence and rights are identical. Clinicians often wish to make a distinction between acts of procreation in which they have had no or only minimal involvement (prescribing clomiphene or advising on the 'fertile period' for example) and identically motivated acts which require high levels of medical and technological input. It could be argued that the existence of the resulting child is just as much or as little the responsibility of the clinician irrespective of their level of involvement.

The Warnock report of 1984, which gave rise to the Human Fertilisation and Embryology Act of 1990, considered the issue of the post-mortem use of gametes and expressed grave misgivings because this use may 'give rise to profound psychological problems for the child and the mother' . However, the report made no direct recommendation for action, stating instead that 'Posthumous use of gametes is a practice which we feel should be actively discouraged'. The Act did not prohibit the retrieval and storage of gametes but required the consent of the source of gametes before they could be stored. It was this aspect of the law that in 1998 prevented Diane Blood being treated in the United Kingdom with sperm that had been illegally

obtained from her dying husband, and equally illegally stored. The European Court allowed the 'export' of the sperm to Belgium, where she was successfully treated and gave birth to two sons.

Issues that arise in the area of posthumous reproduction focus on intention and consent. When there is known intention and legal consent matters may be straightforward, although the requirement for other parties, including the ART team to be involved, raises the possibility that individuals could be frustrated in their intention by other parties' reluctance to cooperate. When intention is merely implied or the only evidence of the deceased's intention is the testimony of a third party with an interest in the outcome, then the issue is more difficult. The recent case in which cryopreserved oocytes, taken from a young cancer victim, were allowed to be exported to America to be fertilised with donor sperm with the intention that the dead girl's mother should act as a surrogate happened in spite of the absence of formally obtained written consent.

12.8.2 Posthumous Children

In general, the law does suggest that the interests of the deceased may be considered to end with their death. It would allow a man, while still alive, to veto extraction of his sperm post-mortem so that his widow could use it in an ICSI cycle she planned to undertake. However, as a society we place enormous emphasis on a legal and moral duty to respect the expressed or even implied wishes of deceased individuals. I may feel very strongly that my uncle was mistaken in leaving his fortune to his local donkey sanctuary, but unless I can show that undue influence was brought to bear on him, I have no chance in law of overturning his will. Similarly there was a case of a widow who, because her late husband had stipulated so in his will, felt morally obliged to have the frozen embryos that she had generated with him transferred to her womb even though she really did not wish to become pregnant, let alone posthumously so.

However much importance we may attach to a deceased person's wishes, I would contend that society does not usually expect them to be allowed to trump the wishes of those who are still alive. We effectively give next of kin the right to have all the transplantable bits of the departed (or departing) loved one for altruistic reasons. And we are ready to accept the next of kin's claim the person associated with the brain-dead body in question was in favour of organ donation.

However, when the issue is one of harvesting gametes it is not at all clear that the wishes of the next of kin carry such authority. We may be deeply sympathetic to the childless widow who wants her late husband's sperm to be retrieved for her future use, but could other family members have claims too? An only child could feel very strongly that he didn't want some posthumous siblings created with whom he would have to share both his mother and his inheritance.

A chilling American example was a woman whose son had suffered catastrophic brain damage as a result of playing Russian roulette with a loaded pistol. On finding his body she called her local ART centre to extract some sperm, before she called the police. Her plan was to find a woman who would act as a surrogate mother for 'her' grandchild. In an equally macabre incident (also in the United States) two teenage sweethearts were fatally injured in a car accident. Both sets of parents wanted to have their children's gametes harvested. They hoped that, with the help of a surrogate mother, they might one day have the grandchildren they had expected their children to produce by more conventional means.

Appeal is often made to the 'welfare of the child' as the means of deciding whether a proposed course of action using ART techniques is valid and appropriate. The welfare of the child who may be born as a result of treatment is regarded by many as the central and most important tenet expressed in the Human Fertilisation and Embryology Act. However, this appeal to the welfare of the posthumous child who may be born if the treatment is successful in achieving a healthy pregnancy is philosophically untenable. A posthumous child may certainly wish that he had been conceived in a more conventional way and he had a father to play football with, but unless his distress at his origins is so great that he genuinely wished to have never been born, he surely has a strong retrospective interest in the application of the technology that engineered his birth.

Society of course also has legitimate interest in this issue and may rightly be charged with a responsibility of ensuring that human beings are not created merely to satisfy the sad cravings of lonely widows or to fulfil the dynastic ambitions of dead tyrants. Clinicians working in the field of ART should similarly be concerned with judgments that have implications for the allocation of scarce resources. In the United

Kingdom, in which public funding of ART is severely and inequitably limited and where all health resources are subject to rationing, the right of access to specialist techniques to achieve posthumous reproduction appears to enjoy appropriately low priority. We may need to consider whether this judgment should be made in an NHS or private medical context. Nevertheless, as long as it continues to be true that many spontaneous conceptions are either unplanned or initially unwanted it seems difficult to justify placing insurmountable legal obstacles in the way of those who actually wish to conceive and have legitimate access to gametes with which so to do.

12.8.3 Controversies in 'Social' or 'Elective' Egg Freezing

Women who wish to freeze their eggs for their own future use face many hurdles. The technique is presented as being relatively unsuccessful, but with vitrification of oocytes and the experience of frozen donor egg banks it is clear that 'young' frozen eggs have a similar reproductive potential to 'fresh' eggs when thawed, fertilised and transferred as blastocysts.

Many recent surveys have shown that women who seek 'social' egg freezing are not doing so because they have other life goals and wish therefore to delay motherhood, but because they have a highly conventional view of parenthood and because they want to have the opportunity to become a mother in a supportive, long-term relationship. It is important that 'social' freezing is not presented as a 'guaranteed' insurance against age-related infertility, but for women who want the chance to be 'genetic' mothers, it may represent an option that they wish to take.

'Social' egg freezing developed from work to preserve the fertility of young women undergoing potentially sterilising chemotherapy, surgery or radiotherapy. In practice, the distinction between 'social' and medical freezing is increasingly difficult to maintain, as significant gynaecological pathologies such as endometriosis or a strong family history of premature menopause may also represent a compelling argument for oocyte freezing for fertility preservation. In the United Kingdom, women diagnosed with premature and irreversible infertility may have their eggs frozen for 55 years. The passage of time is just as destructive as chemotherapy to a woman's fertility prospects and yet the legislation for 'social' freezers in the United Kingdom limits the storage period of their eggs to only 10 years. This time limit is recognised to be arbitrary and unscientific and it has the paradoxical effect of encouraging women to delay having their eggs frozen beyond the point at which the process is most effective.

There is sparse evidence about the 'usage' rate of socially frozen eggs, as most data sets do not distinguish between the various different reasons for which the eggs have been frozen. It is, however, the experience of UK centres that have pioneered 'social' egg freezing that women either return within a few years to use their eggs (often with donor sperm), or never return at all because presumably they have achieved a natural pregnancy, had successful conventional fertility treatment or they have never met a suitable partner to parent with.

'Social' egg freezers represent a particularly challenging group of patients, partly because they are often facing severe disappointment that they are not in a position to start a family in a conventional relationship and they are understandably anxious about undergoing a medical procedure that carries no guarantees of a successful outcome. Supportive counselling is absolutely vital at all stages of their treatment cycle.

12.9 Donor Gametes: Ethical Issues for Donors, Recipients and Their Offspring

Donor gametes (eggs and sperm) clearly have an equal genetic contribution to make to the creation of an embryo and hence to a potential person, but the very different problems of procurement should not be allowed to overshadow the fact that the ethical issues for donors and recipients are identical.

Until the end of donor anonymity was enacted in law in 2005, gamete donors were guaranteed lifelong anonymity in the United Kingdom and this was thought to be a factor in encouraging young men to become sperm donors. This decision to end anonymity followed a prolonged period of review and public consultation. When fertility clinics were consulted, the majority were opposed because of concerns that it would deter donors at a time when there was already a shortage of donor sperm, and that the removal of anonymity would have no effect on secrecy, as many parents never tell their children that a donor was involved in their conception. This is not to underestimate the distress of donor-conceived people who

know of their origins but are unable to find out any useful, let alone identifiable, information about their genetic parent.

The incidence of non-paternity (where a child is not the offspring of his or her putative father) has been estimated as being between 2% and 12% in the general population and as high as 25% where paternity testing is undertaken because suspicions have been raised. An MP on the Select Committee of Science and Technology that reviewed the legislation actually suggested that all newborns should be DNA fingerprinted to ensure that everyone could exercise their fundamental *right* to know their true genetic identity.

One aspect of the ending of anonymity that was inherent in the new legislation was the degree of asymmetry in available information introduced between a donor's 'own' children and their 'biological' siblings and half-siblings.

Donor sperm, egg or embryo conceived individuals can apply to the HFEA 'Opening the Register' team for identifiable information about their donors, *if* they know they are donor conceived, at the age of 18, or earlier if they are considering marriage and wish to confirm they are not related to their intended partner. This enquiry will also supply information about siblings and half-siblings if any. However, although donors can be told the outcome of their donations (restricted to number, year of birth and gender), they cannot have any further information for their own children. If they tell their children that they have half-siblings (or in the case of embryo donation, full siblings) and those donor conceived offspring never try to establish contact, then these young people may be left with a 'gap' in their genetic record, which was part of the reason why anonymity was ended. However, if the donor does not reveal their donation history to their own children and the family is informed that one or more 18-year-olds is wanting to make contact, that could have harmful repercussions in terms of family trust.

Modern technology in the form of direct-to-consumer (DTC) DNA testing and ancestry tracing may already be undermining the theoretical guarantees of anonymity that donors were offered prior to 2004. People may buy DTC tests for a variety of purposes but may discover that they are donor conceived and there are DNA-based voluntary contact registers that may allow them to identify both their donor and any siblings.

The current advice is that clinical teams should provide support, guidance and information on the availability and implications of genetic ancestry testing and the lack of control over identity that an individual may have if a blood relation undergoes testing.

12.9.1 Surrogacy

Surrogacy, or at least 'straight' surrogacy, where the birth mother is also the genetic mother, may claim to be one of the oldest forms of fertility treatment, as it has been practiced since Biblical times. However, most surrogacy arrangements in the United Kingdom involve 'host' or 'gestational' surrogacy where the surrogate mother has no direct genetic link to the child who will be born and will become the legal offspring of the genetic or 'intended parents' (IPs) who have provided the gametes in an IVF treatment.

There are many reasons why IPs turn to surrogacy:

- Recurrent miscarriage
- Repeated failure of IVF treatment
- Premature menopause, often as a result of cancer treatment
- A hysterectomy or an absent or abnormal uterus
- A serious risk to health that may result from pregnancy
- LGBT+ parents wanting to create a family.

Britain was in advance of many other jurisdictions in legislating to legalise surrogacy, mainly as a result of a media and professional outcry in the 1980s following the 'Baby Cotton' case in which Kim Cotton admitted to being paid to bear babies for other women. Many European countries outlaw surrogacy, believing that it encourages 'child abandonment', and the establishment of 'baby farms' in developing countries, where poor women act as host surrogates for Western couples, has rightly raised issues of exploitation and the commodification of reproduction.

In straight surrogacy (also known as full or traditional) the surrogate provides her own eggs to achieve the pregnancy. The intended father, in either a heterosexual or male same-sex relationship, provides a sperm sample for conception through either self-insemination at home or artificial insemination with the help of a fertility clinic. If either the surrogate or intended father has fertility issues, then embryos may also be created in vitro and transferred into the uterus of the surrogate.

Although surrogacy is legal in the United Kingdom, surrogacy arrangements are not enforceable in law. The Surrogacy Arrangements Act 1985 makes it clear that it is an offence to advertise that you are seeking a surrogate or are a potential surrogate looking for IPs. It is also an offence under that Act to arrange or negotiate a surrogacy arrangement as a commercial enterprise; however, there are a number of non-profit organisations (also known as 'altruistic') that lawfully assist potential surrogates and IPs to navigate their surrogacy.

The surrogate (and, if she is married or in a civil partnership, her consenting spouse or civil partner) will be the legal parents of the child at birth. Following the birth, there is a legal process – the parental order process – to transfer legal parenthood from the surrogate to the IPs. To apply for a parental order and transfer legal parenthood, at least one of the IPs must be genetically related to the baby. Single people/parents cannot currently apply for parental orders in surrogacy cases, but the government intends to introduce legislation that, if passed, would enable them to do so.

The parental order criteria are strict and indicate the level of anxiety that surrounds the whole area. There have been cases in which mothers of women who need a surrogate have effectively 'given birth to their own grandchild' by having an embryo created from their daughter and son-in-law's gametes transferred to their uterus. It is possible that the developing success of 'womb transplants' from both cadaveric and living-related donors may reduce the demand for surrogacy, but there is little evidence at present.

As with all issues arising in assisted conception, the welfare of the child who may be born (or a child who may be affected by that birth) is pre-eminent. In surrogacy arrangements, it is particularly clear that the information imparted to the child may be vital. The inevitably close relationship that develops between IPs and the surrogate mother (and partner) should encourage an open and honest explanation of the child's origins, but some IPs come to see the process as a form of 'pre-implantation adoption' and do not wish to accord their surrogate a role beyond birth.

In ethical terms it is difficult to justify a distinction between the role of the 'straight' or the 'host' surrogate. It is possible that a host surrogate mother may feel less 'attached' to her newborn if she has no genetic link, but IPs should be sensitive to the needs of their surrogate and her children (who may perceive that they have lost a potential sibling).

12.10 'Designing Babies': Balancing Autonomy with Welfare of the Child and Societal Concerns

In the developed world, the greatest cause of early death and disability is genetic disease and so it is clearly tempting to consider the application of preimplantation genetic diagnosis (PGD) as an adjunct to contemporary fertility treatment. PGD is a procedure used prior to embryo implantation to identify genetic defects within embryos. These could be 'expected' where PGD is being carried out because the prospective parents are aware that they carry deleterious genes (i.e. both are CF carriers) or because there is an increased risk of aneuploidy due to advanced maternal age or history of recurrent miscarriage. A procedure which allows prospective parents to embark on a pregnancy confident that their baby will not be affected by a lethal genetic disease or that the normally high age–related risk of miscarriage due to aneuploidy has been significantly reduced would seem to be universally acceptable.

One could even envisage couples who do not *need* IVF to conceive choosing to undergo ART so that their potential children could be 'screened' for rare genetic diseases. Some diseases have variable penetrance and some only generate symptoms in middle or older age. Many would perceive the use of PGD for sex-selection as an unacceptable application of the PGD technology, but gender-based selective termination is widely practised and would seem even less ethically acceptable.

A significant ethical issue in embryo screening and embryo selection relates to decisions about what qualifies as a sufficiently serious or likely genetic anomaly that it is acceptable to screen for it and not transfer affected embryos. Some communities such as those with congenital deafness or achondroplastic dwarfism have claimed a right to screen *for* genetic characteristics that many would consider to be deleterious.

Often described as a 'slippery slope', it is very likely that many physical and even intellectual characteristics may soon be identifiable in PGD screening and then it may prove impossible to put this eugenic genie back in the bottle.

12.11 Conclusion

The field of assisted reproduction remains one of the most rapidly evolving branches of medicine and perhaps, what is most remarkable – and the source of its most contentious ethical dilemmas – is that it involves arguably more significant outcomes than any other branches. In ART we are not just saving lives (the pinnacle of oncology therapy or transplant surgery), we are actually *creating* lives with all the implications that entails for the individual, the family and society.

Developments such as CRISPR (clustered regularly interspaced short palindromic repeats), cadaveric womb transplants for transgender women and pre-pubescent testicular xeno-transplants for boys requiring sterilising chemotherapies have moved our field from the realm of science fiction to the theoretically and actually possible. It is vital that philosophers who speculate on the ethical challenges of our field are very well informed about what we can and are doing, and it is equally important that doctors and scientists consider the potential ethical implications of their work. As with the (near) universal ban on human cloning, we don't need to do something just because we can. Inevitably, we will be leading and informing political and public opinion about these contentious and challenging issues. Arguably, we must stay out in front – but not too far.

Further Reading

Beauchamp T, Childress J. *Principles of biomedical ethics*, 4th ed. New York: Oxford University Press; 1994.

Cameron C, Williamson R. Is there an ethical difference between preimplantation genetic diagnosis and abortion? *J Med Ethics*. 2003;29:90–2.

Lockwood GM. Social egg freezing: the prospect of reproductive 'immortality' or a dangerous delusion? *Reprod BioMed Online*. 2011; 23:334–40.

Lockwood MJ. The moral status of the human embryo: implications for IVF. *RBMOnline*. 2005;10(Suppl 1): 17–20.

Savulescu J. Procreative beneficence: why we should select the best children. *Bioethics* 2001;15(5/6).

13

Evidence-Based Reproductive Medicine

Siladitya Bhattacharya

13.1 Introduction

Evidence-based medicine (EBM) is the conscientious, explicit and judicious use of current best evidence to make clinical decisions [1], while integrating clinical expertise, experience and awareness of an individual patient's preferences. Although this process of decision-making might sound laborious and contrived, much of it occurs intuitively in day-to-day clinical practice. EBM in everyday clinical practice can be challenging but, with the appropriate mindset, it is well within the capability of the average clinician entirely feasible and, given the pace of progress in reproductive medicine, increasingly, an essential part of effective care. It is, however, contingent on the ability to use digital technology to search the literature and use basic appraisal skills to judge the quality and relevance of available evidence. EBM demands clinical knowledge, both in terms of informing the parameters for a successful literature search as well as deciding whether and how the results match the patient's clinical state, predicament and preferences. Evidence-based guidelines can overcome the necessity for repetitive individual searches but are unable to overcome lack of basic subject-specific knowledge and poor decision-making processes or treatment skills.

Any clinical encounter generates questions about diagnostic and treatment strategies as well as concerns about side effects. The aim of a fertility consultation should be to discuss a set of options as a basis for joint decision-making, incorporating the preferences and values of both partners. For example, a couple presenting with unexplained infertility may wish to know whether they should undergo active treatment with superovulation and intrauterine insemination (SO-IUI) or in vitro fertilisation (IVF). This will require knowledge about their chances of success without treatment, the effectiveness of both treatments and expectations around the time required to conceive.

13.2 Using EBM to Inform Clinical Decision-Making

In practice, it is important to approach clinical questions through an EBM lens using a series of sequential steps (see Figure 13.1).

13.2.1 Framing a Structured Question

The first step in EBM is to convert a clinical question – for example, 'What is the best way to manage unexplained infertility?' – into a series of specific questions

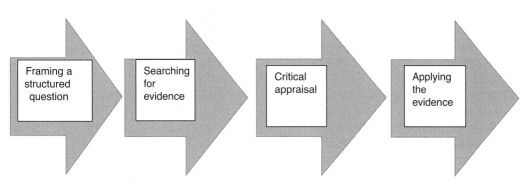

| Framing a structured question | Searching for evidence | Critical appraisal | Applying the evidence |

Figure 13.1 Sequential steps in approaching clinical questions through an EBM lens.

Table 13.1 Asking a question

Clinical question	EBM question
Should a couple with unexplained infertility be offered superovulation and intrauterine insemination?	In couples with unexplained infertility, how does superovulation with IUI compare with no treatment or IVF?
Population	Couples with unexplained infertility
Intervention	Superovulation and intrauterine insemination
Comparator	No treatment (expectant management) or IVF
Outcome	Live births per couple
Design	Randomised trial

by defining key components such as the population of interest, the proposed intervention, the comparison – that is, no treatment or another intervention, the outcome of interest and the type of research design which is best suited to answering the question. For example, for the earlier question the ideal type of evidence is provided by randomised trials or, even better, by systematic reviews based on them. Table 13.1 shows examples of how this can be achieved in different areas of reproductive medicine.

13.2.2 Searching the Literature

A comprehensive search of the literature can be a detailed and time-consuming process which can be made much simpler by following a few basic rules. A hierarchical approach aimed at identifying clinical practice guidelines and evidence-based reviews rather than primary research papers can be helpful, provided they are relevant and of high quality. National bodies such as the National Institute for Health and Care Excellence (NICE) in the United Kingdom as well as professional organisations such as the European Society for Human Reproduction and Embryology (ESHRE), the American Society for Reproductive Medicine (ASRM), the British Fertility Society (BFS) and the Royal College of Obstetricians and Gynaecologists (RCOG) generate guidelines which are periodically updated. Where high-quality evidence-based guidelines are unavailable, clinicians

need to search for good quality systematic reviews, or in their absence, primary studies. Databases such as Medline and PubMed can be interrogated for systematic reviews or primary studies. A systematic search needs keywords matched to the medical subject heading terms and combined using Boolean operators such as 'and', 'or' and so forth.

13.2.2.1 Systematic Reviews

A systematic review uses prespecified methods to locate and appraise data and, where appropriate, undertake formal aggregation of quantitative data (meta-analysis). Well-conducted systematic reviews are preferable to individual studies as sources of high-quality evidence because single studies may be unrepresentative and lack the power to provide definitive answers to some questions. Inconsistent results across different publications on the same research question can be explored, and the ability to pool data allows greater precision around estimation of effects of interventions. Systematic reviews of randomised trials are considered to represent the highest quality of evidence on the effectiveness of medical and surgical treatments as well as more complex interventions such as IVF. Systematic reviews of observational studies are becoming increasingly more common, and may be the only source of evidence in situations where randomised trials do not exist or where randomisation is not feasible but results of meta-analyses need careful interpretation, as they are prone to bias.

13.2.2.2 Randomised Trials

A randomised trial can overcome many of the risks of bias associated with observational studies and provide convincing evidence to inform the choice of effective treatments. Random treatment allocation ensures that the two populations receiving different treatments are similar in terms of characteristics which could affect the results of treatment. Thus, any differences in outcomes can be assumed to be genuinely due to the intervention. Non-randomised studies with control arms may offer some information about effective treatments but are prone to confounding by patient characteristics which can influence non-random allocation of treatments. Not all randomised trials are of similar quality and some can be compromised by poor study design, execution or data analysis. A clear consort flow (Figure 13.2) is an essential component of a well reported trial which provides useful information about methodological rigour.

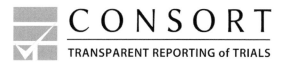

CONSORT

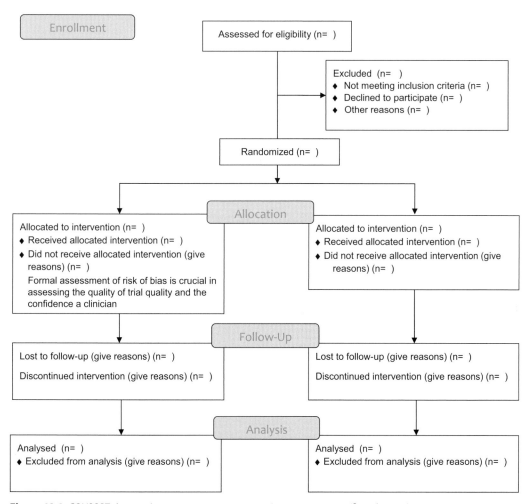

Figure 13.2 CONSORT diagram (www.consort-statement.org/consort-statement/flow-diagram)

A traditional problem associated with infertility trials has been the multiplicity of outcomes and the way in which they are defined – something which will hopefully be addressed by the adoption of core outcome sets [2].

13.2.2.3 Observational Studies

Data from observational studies are useful in answering questions regarding the association between cause and effect, that is, exposure to smoking and its reproductive consequences. Thus, they are helpful in aiding clinicians to make decisions regarding diagnosis, causality and prognosis. In addition, as most randomised trials have relatively short periods of follow-up unlimited sample sizes larger observational studies population-based with long-term follow-up data can be useful in identifying side-effects of drugs over time. Where trials do not exist or are not feasible because of ethical considerations, observational studies may be the only source of data on the effectiveness of interventions.

13.2.2.4 Diagnostic Test Accuracy Studies

The quality and usefulness of investigations are usually assessed by means of diagnostic accuracy studies which measure sensitivity, specificity and predictive values (Figure 13.3). Patients can test positive or negative for any condition. A common way of evaluating the quality of tests is to determine the proportions of patients with normal and abnormal test results which were identified correctly. Sensitivity reflects the proportion of true positives while specificity represents the proportion of true negatives that are correctly identified by a test.

An estimate of the probability that the test will give us the correct diagnosis is better explored by means of positive and negative predictive values for a test. The former represents the proportion of patients with positive test results who are correctly diagnosed, while the latter reflects the proportion of patients with a negative test who are accurately identified. Predictive value is strongly influenced by the prevalence of the condition being tested for. If the prevalence of the disease is very low, the positive predictive value will be poor even if the sensitivity and specificity for a test are high. In population-based screening using serum anti-müllerian hormone, it is inevitable that many women with a positive test will be false positive. The ratio of the probability of getting a positive test result if the patient genuinely had a condition with the corresponding probability if she were healthy is the likelihood ratio – calculated as sensitivity/(1– specificity). The likelihood ratio indicates the value of the test for increasing certainty about a positive diagnosis. In general, the higher the likelihood ratio of an abnormal test the greater is its usefulness; for example, values of 10 or more suggest that the test could be extremely useful while a value of 1 suggests that it is useless. For a negative test a likelihood ratio of 0.1 or less suggests that it is useful while a value of 1 indicates that it is not.

13.2.3 Critical Appraisal of the Literature

The quality of evidence acquired by means of a literature search needs to be assessed through a process of critical appraisal. This can be done using a number of tools such as those available from the Centre for Evidence based Medicine (www.cebm.net/2014/06/critical-appraisal/) or the critical appraisal skills programme (https://casp-uk.net/). Any appraisal of the quality of a systematic review should include assessment of the credibility of the methods used, assessment of the risk of bias and confidence in the effect estimates. Clinicians also need to be confident that the population studied is similar to that of patients in whom an intervention is proposed (directness). In addition to being effective, it is necessary for a treatment to be affordable, culturally acceptable and provide benefits which outweigh harm.

While systematic reviews can often provide high-quality evidence based on results from a number of individual studies, not all are of similar quality and blind acceptance of results from meta-analyses can lead to poor clinical practice. Standards such as the Preferred Reporting Items for Systematic Reviews and Meta-Analyses (PRISMA) statement [4] have described best practice in terms of undertaking and reporting systematic reviews. The Cochrane handbook contains guidance for those undertaking systematic reviews but does not include a critical appraisal tool for reviewers. The quality of systematic reviews can be formally evaluated using a number of practical tools available from the Centre for Evidence Based Medicine (CEBM) www.cebm.net/category/eb

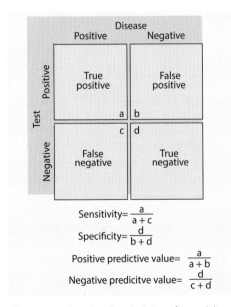

Figure 13.3 Template for calculation of test validity.

Source: Uses and abuses of screening tests. Grimes DA, Schulz KF. *Lancet.* 2002;359(9309):881–4 [3]

m-resources/tools/critically-appraising-the-evidence/ which assist clinicians in evaluating the quality of evidence by assessing the validity of the results, methodological quality and relevance, that is, how likely it is that the intended population shares the same characteristic as those of the research subjects. AMSTAR2 has been recently developed as a comprehensive tool for assessing the quality of systematic reviews of randomised or non-randomised studies and assisting medical practitioners to base clinical decisions on real-world observational evidence [5].

Assessment of risk of bias is a key element of all systematic reviews. The most commonly used tool is the Cochrane risk of bias tool, which was introduced in 2008. The revised version [6] considers bias in five domains (see Table 13.2) to determine whether there is 'low risk of bias', 'some concerns' or 'high risk of bias'.

These in turn lead to an overall risk of bias judgement for the result being assessed such that meta-analyses can be stratified according to risk of bias (see Table 13.3).

13.2.4 Applying the Evidence

The final step in evidence-based medicine is implementation of the identified evidence in clinical practice. In practice this can be complex, as it needs consideration of several issues including relevance,

Table 13.2 Version 2 of the Cochrane risk-of-bias assessment tool for randomised trials: Bias domains, signalling questions, response options, and risk-of-bias judgments

Bias domain and signalling question*	Response options		
	Lower risk of bias	Higher risk of bias	Other
Bias arising from the randomisation process			
1.1 Was the allocation sequence random?	Y/PY	N/PN	NI
1.2 Was the allocation sequence concealed until participants were enrolled and assigned to interventions?	Y/PY	N/PN	NI
1.3 Did baseline differences between intervention groups suggest a problem with the randomisation process?	N/PN	Y/PY	NI
Risk-of-bias judgment (low/high/some concerns)			
Optional: What is the predicted direction of bias arising from the randomisation process?			
Bias due to deviations from intended interventions			
2.1 Were participants aware of their assigned intervention during the trial?	N/PN	Y/PY	NI
2.2 Were carers and people delivering the interventions aware of participants' assigned intervention during the trial?	N/PN	Y/PY	NI
2.3 If Y/PY/NI to 2.1 or 2.2: Were there deviations from the intended intervention that arose because of the trial context?	N/PN	Y/PY	NA/NI
2. A If Y/PY/NI to 2.3: Were these deviations likely to have affected the outcome?	N/PN	Y/PY	NA/NI
2.5 If Y/PY to 2.4: Were these deviations from intended intervention balanced between groups?	Y/PY	N/PN	NA/NI
2.6 Was an appropriate analysis used to estimate the effect of assignment to intervention?	Y/PY	N/PN	NI
2.7 If N/PN/NI to 2.6: Was there potential for a substantial impact (on the result) of the failure to analyse participants in the group to which they were randomised?	N/PN	Y/PY	NA/NI
Risk-of-bias judgment (low/high/some concerns)			
Optional: What is the predicted direction of bias due to deviations from intended interventions?			
Bias due to missing outcome data			
3.1 Were data for this outcome available for all, or nearly all, participants randomised?	Y/PY	N/PN	NI
3.2 If N/PN/NI to 3.1: Is there evidence that the result was not biased by missing	Y/PY	N/PN	NA

Table 13.2 (cont.)

Bias domain and signalling question*	Response options		
	Lower risk of bias	Higher risk of bias	Other
3.3 If N/PN to 3.2: Could missingness in the outcome depend on its true value?	N/PN	Y/PY	NA/NI
3.4 If Y/PY/NI to 3.3: Is it likely that missingness in the outcome depended on its true value?	N/PN	Y/PY	NA/NI
Risk-of-bias judgment (low/high/some concerns)			
Optional: What is the predicted direction of bias due to missing outcome data?			
Bias in measurement of the outcome			
4.1 Was the method of measuring the outcome inappropriate?	N/PN	Y/PY	NI
4.2 Could measurement or ascertainment of the outcome have differed between intervention groups?	N/PN	Y/PY	NI
4.3 If N/PN/NI to 4.1 and 4.2: Were outcome assessors aware of the intervention received by study participants?	N/PN	Y/PY	NI
4.4 If Y/PY/NI to 4.3: Could assessment of the outcome have been influenced by knowledge of intervention received?	N/PN	Y/PY	NA/NI
4.5 If Y/PY/NI to 4.4: Is it likely that assessment of the outcome was influenced by knowledge of intervention received?	N/PN	Y/PY	NA/NI
Risk-of-bias judgment (low/high/some concerns)			
Optional: What is the predicted direction of bias in measurement of the outcome?			
Bias in selection of the reported result			
5.1 Were the data that produced this result analysed in accordance with a prespecified analysis plan that was finalised before unblinded outcome data were available for analysis?	Y/PY	N/PN	NI
Is the numerical result being assessed likely to have been selected, on the basis of the results, from:			
5.2 … multiple eligible outcome measurements (e.g. scales, definitions, time points) within the outcome domain?	N/PN	Y/PY	NI
5.3 … multiple eligible analyses of the data?	N/PN	Y/PY	NI
Risk-of-bias judgment (low/high/some concerns)			
Optional: What is the predicted direction bias due to selection of the reported results?			
Overall bias			
Risk-of-bias judgment (low/high/some concerns)			
Optional: What is the overall predicted direction of bias for this outcome?			

Y = yes; PY = probably yes; PN = probably no; N = no; NA = not applicable; NI = no information.
'Signalling questions for bias due to deviations from intended interventions relate to the effect of assignment to intervention.
From ref. [6].

quality, balance of benefit versus harm and affordability.

13.2.4.1 Relevance or Generalisability

This refers to a judgment as to whether the results of a study or studies are applicable to a clinician's own practice. It is important to use reasonable flexibility, coupled with clinical judgment to inform any conclusions. For example, how likely is it that the results of IVF trials in women under 38 could be relevant to a 42-year-old woman contemplating assisted reproduction? Although the patient in question may not have been eligible for the original trials there is no reason to believe that the direction of effect should be any different, although the margin of benefit, that is, the absolute improvement of a treatment, might be smaller than seen in the aggregated data from trials on younger women.

Table 13.3 Approach to reaching an overall risk-of-bias judgment for a specific result

Overall risk-of-bias judgment	Criteria
Low risk of bias	The study is judged to be at low risk of bias for all domains for this result
Some concerns	The study is judged to raise some concerns in at least one domain for this result, but not to be at high risk of bias for any domain
High risk of bias	The study is judged to be at high risk of bias in at least one domain for this result, or the study is judged to have some concerns for multiple domains in a way that substantially lowers confidence in the result

From ref. [6].

13.2.4.2 Overall Quality of Evidence

How do we evaluate the body of evidence to decide whether it is fit for purpose? The considerations which need to inform our judgement include validity, precision and local relevance. The GRADE system assesses evidence in terms of four levels: high, moderate, low and very low [7]. Data from randomised trials are initially rated as high-quality evidence but can be downgraded on the basis of the following criteria: study limitations, inconsistency of results, indirectness of evidence, imprecision and reporting bias. Conversely, observational studies are assumed to be of lower quality but can be upgraded if the effect size is very large, there is a dose–response effect or if all plausible biases would likely decrease the magnitude of the effect.

In terms of making the final decision, there are several factors which influence our strength of conviction about any evidence-based decision (Table 13.4).

13.3 Guidelines

Clinical practice guidelines are now a common feature of clinical practice. They are expected to improve patient outcomes through a culture of medical practice which is consistent, effective and efficient – but defining the quality of guidelines is not easy. Good guidelines need to be scientifically valid, usable and reliable. In the absence of data which can attest to these attributes, users have attempted to access information on whether the guideline producers have attempted to minimise all the biases associated with guideline development and reporting. The AGREE instrument is designed to assess the process of guideline development and how well this process is reported [8]. It does not assess the clinical content of the guideline or the quality of evidence that underpins the recommendations. The criteria for high-quality clinical guidelines are shown in Box 13.1. Over the years, the process of guideline development has evolved to a point where the discerning clinician can identify reliable and relevant guidance which is able to demonstrate focus, methodological rigour, clarity and editorial independence.

Apart from the obvious elements of effectiveness backed up with precise and valid data, many successful treatments have side effects and a joint decision may need to be made with the patient as to whether any anticipated benefits are outweighed by potential side-effects. This, along with considerations of cost might influence clinical decisions. Implementation of evidence in the public domain has often been slow – partly because of how benefits, side effects and costs are often charged intuitively or perceived very differently in different clinical contexts and funding frameworks. When there are several treatment options with comparable benefits, there is a strong case for offering the patient these choices and involving them actively in the decision-making process. It has been shown that this may actually increase the effectiveness of the treatment itself. Decision analysis, which provides an intellectual framework for an explicit decision-making algorithm, and computerised decision support systems are approaches that might be considered within the framework of digital medicine.

13.4 Conclusion

Evidence-based medicine is an integral part of clinical practice but can be challenging due to the sheer volume of published research, the time needed to search the literature and the skills necessary to critically review the quality of the available evidence. High-quality clinical guidelines have made the task of the clinicians somewhat easier but there are many of them and it is necessary to use some of the available tools to assess their quality. Finally, clinicians need to be aware of the importance of accommodating the needs of their patients as well as the demands of their health care delivery system.

Table 13.4 Rating overall confidence in the results of a review

High
- No or one non-critical weakness: The systematic review provides an accurate and comprehensive summary of the results of the available studies that address the question of interest.

Moderate
- More than one non-critical weakness[a]: The systematic review has more than one weakness but no critical flaws. It may provide an accurate summary of the results of the available studies that were included in the review.

Low
- One critical flaw with or without non-critical weaknesses: The review has a critical flaw and may not provide an accurate and comprehensive summary of the available studies that address the question of interest.

Critically low
- More than one critical flaw with or without non-critical weaknesses: The review has more than one critical flaw and should not be relied on to provide an accurate and comprehensive summary of the available studies.

*Multiple non-critical weaknesses may diminish confidence in the review and it may be appropriate to move the overall appraisal down from moderate to low confidence.

From ref. [5]

Box 13.1 Criteria of High-Quality Clinical Practice Guidelines

1. Scope and purpose

Contain a specific statement about the overall objective(s), clinical questions, and describes the target population.

2. Stakeholder involvement

Provide information about the composition, discipline, and relevant expertise of the guideline development group and involve patients in their development. They also clearly define the target users and have been piloted prior to publication.

3. Rigour of development

Provide detailed information on the search strategy, the inclusion and exclusion criteria for selecting the evidence, and the methods used to formulate the recommendations. The recommandations are explicitlylinked to the supporting evidene and there is a discussion of the health benefits, side effect, and risk. They have been externally reviewed before publication and provide detailed information about the procedure for updating the guideline.

4. Clarity and presentation

Contain specific recommendations on appropriate patient care and consider different possible options. The key recommendations are easily found. A summary document and patients' leaflets are provided.

5. Applicability

Discuss the organisational changes and cost implications of applying the recommendations and present review criteria for monitoring the use of the guidelines.

6. Editorial independene

Include an explicit statement that the views or interests of the funding body have not influenced the final recommendations. Members of the guideline group have declared possible conflicts of interest.

Source: AGREE Collaboration. *Quality and Safety in Health Care* 2003.

References

1. Sackett DL, Rosenberg WM, Gray JA, Haynes RB, Richardson WS. Evidence based medicine: what it is and what it isn't. *BMJ*. 1996;**312**(7023):71–2.

2. Duffy JMN, Bhattacharya S, Curtis C, Evers JLH, Farquharson RG, Franik S, et al. COMMIT: Core Outcomes Measures for Infertility Trials. A protocol developing, disseminating and implementing a core outcome set for infertility. *Hum Reprod Open*. 2018(**3**): hoy007. DOI: 10.1093/hropen/hoy007. eCollection 2018.

3. Grimes DA, Schulz KF. Uses and abuses of screening tests. *Lancet*. 2002 Mar 9;**359**(9309):881–4. Review. Erratum in: Lancet. 2008;371(9629):1998.

4. Moher D, Liberati A, Tetzlaff J, Altman DG; PRISMA Group. Preferred reporting items for systematic reviews and meta-analyses: the PRISMA statement. *Ann Intern Med*. 2009;**151**(4):264–9, W64. Epub 2009 Jul 20.

5. Shea BJ, Reeves BC, Wells G, Thuku M, Hamel C, Moran J, AMSTAR 2: a critical appraisal tool for systematic reviews that include randomised or non-randomised studies of healthcare interventions, or both. *BMJ*. 2017;**358**:j4008. DOI: 10.1136/bmj.j4008.

6. Sterne JAC, Savović J, Page MJ, Elbers RG, Blencowe NS, Boutron I, et al. RoB 2: a revised tool for assessing risk of bias in randomised trials. *BMJ*. 2019;**366**:l4898. DOI: 10.1136/bmj.l4898.

7. Guyatt GH, Oxman AD, Vist GE, Kunz R, Falck-Ytter Y, Alonso-Coello P, Schünemann HJ; GRADE Working Group. GRADE: an emerging consensus on rating quality of evidence and strength of recommendations. *BMJ*. 2008;**336**(7650):924–6. DOI: 10.1136/bmj.39489.470347.AD.

8. AGREE Collaboration. Development and validation of an international appraisal instrument for assessing the quality of clinical practice guidelines: the AGREE project. *Qual Saf Health Care*. 2003;**12**(1):18–23.

The Organisation of Services and Quality Assurance in Fertility Practice

Alison McTavish and Mark Hamilton

14.1 Introduction

Following the landmark achievement of the first in vitro fertilisation (IVF) birth in 1978 major advances in the clinical and laboratory techniques in assisted conception practice have widened the scope and efficacy of treatment. These included the refinement of ovarian stimulation protocols, ultrasound guided oocyte retrieval, cryopreservation of surplus embryos, egg donation, surrogacy, intracytoplasmic sperm injection (ICSI), surgical sperm retrieval, in vitro maturation of oocytes, preimplantation genetic testing of embryos and the use of gonadotropin-releasing hormone antagonists.

In the United Kingdom, these advances took place within a regulatory framework administered by the Human Fertilisation and Embryology Authority (HFEA) empowered through an Act of Parliament. Oversight and regulation within the burgeoning sector were further moderated by the European Tissues and Cells Directive (EUTCD) in 2004. Continued progress in specific areas such as ovarian tissue cryopreservation and transplantation, preimplantation genetic diagnosis and screening and somatic cell nuclear transfer were complemented by a revision of the 1990 Human Fertilisation and Embryology (HFE) Act in 2008.

More recently, elective single embryo transfer, the individualisation of stimulation regimes to maximise outcomes through ovarian reserve testing, the advent of vitrification of eggs and embryos, fertility preservation for young women facing potentially sterilising medical or surgical treatment of cancer and other conditions have expanded the scope of assisted reproductive technologies in the reproductive health care. In the United Kingdom, some 2% of all births are attributable to the use of IVF, with nearly 70,000 treatment cycles across 80 licensed centres. Responding to major laboratory and clinical advances has been a requirement for clinics in an increasingly competitive environment where the client group has high expectations. In the United Kingdom, all licensed IVF centres are required by the HFEA Code of Practice to have a quality management system to ensure a uniform standard of excellence.

This quality-based approach to the delivery of assisted reproductive technology (ART) services has become an integral part of the management of the infertile couple. It underpins a patient-centred approach from first contact, through assessment and diagnostic pathways, first-line treatment and ultimately assisted conception.

This chapter seeks to give an overview of the place of Quality Management in contemporary fertility practice.

14.2 Defining Quality and Success

Providing the best care for patients lies at the heart of good medicine. However, as this book shows, there are many stages in the pathway of fertility treatment, with many stakeholders involved. It is important to establish agreement between patients and professionals on factors which are perceived to be critical in defining the quality of care.

The World Health Organization suggests that a health system should seek to ensure that the following dimensions of quality are considered in the organisation of services:

- Care should be **effective**, predicated on sound evidence, resulting in improved health outcomes addressing the needs of service users.
- Care should be **efficient**, maximising use of resources and avoiding waste.
- Care should be **accessible**, that is, deliverable at an appropriate time in the care pathway and in a place where skills and resources are available to meet the medical need.
- The preferences of users of services should be taken account of in accordance with **patient-centred** principles of care.

- The quality of care should be available on an **equitable** basis, without prejudice relevant to issues such as gender, race, ethnicity, sexual orientation or socio-economic status.
- **Safe** delivery of care minimising risks and harm to users of services is essential.

Service delivery in line with these principles utilises a number of tools to monitor performance against agreed upon standards and these will be considered in more detail.

Quality Management, quality assurance, quality control are quality improvement are terms which are commonly used in this context. It is useful to compare and contrast the meanings of these terms to better understand how they are related.

Quality Management describes the establishment of a system which enables an organisation, in this case a clinic, to provide a standard of service which leads to a consistent level of excellence. This is provided within a culture of continual monitoring of performance and effort to improve the quality and effectiveness of the service. A commonly used resource to facilitate the introduction of quality management is the Quality Management Systems – Requirements ISO 9001:2015.

Quality assurance sets out to maintain a high level of quality by monitoring and recording every stage in a process of care thereby facilitating identification of specific problems associated with an overall reduction in performance. An example of this might be a fall in the expected number of cleavage stage embryos which might develop from normally fertilised eggs within the incubator. The consequence of this could be a reduction in the number of pregnancies and live births resultant from treatment within the centre.

Quality control is the mechanism whereby a clinic monitors specific elements within the process of care which may directly or indirectly impact on the quality of outcome for the patient engaging with the clinical service. This might, for example, include the use of specific equipment to assess the temperature and pH within an incubator used to culture embryos. Problems with either of these variables may be the cause of the embryo cleavage issues alluded to earlier.

Quality improvement describes the responsibility of a clinic to set in place actions with the aim of enhancing outcomes. The clinic might, in response to problems with embryo cleavage, choose to introduce changes in the culture media used in the embryo incubator. Monitoring systems to assess the impact of any change should be in place to provide objective evidence that the adaptation to the protocols used have led to the desired improvement.

14.3 Using a Process Model in the Organisation of Services

The goal in quality management is to enable the provision of a high-quality clinical service, underpinned by evidence, at a standard which is consistent for all patients and customers.

An assessment of the functional needs of the clinic is best achieved through a process model approach (Figure 14.1). This encompasses the three elements of encounter with any organisation: an input, a process and an output. In fertility care, the patient is at the heart of every process.

To demonstrate how this applies in a fertility clinic setting it is best to consider the input in this situation to be the patients referred to the clinic. This might be from general practitioners or hospital colleagues, while some users of the service may self-refer.

Receipt of the referral triggers a *process* of care. This process should be mapped carefully such that each stage may be considered individually and in the context of the overall pathway. A referral would normally encompass consultation, assessment, investigation and treatment by highly trained and adequately equipped staff. A trained multidisciplinary team will be involved in the delivery of care whose members will require access to and possession of facilities, materials and good levels of internal/external communication; they need to provide relevant and understandable information for users of services, and utilise sound clinical methods encompassing knowledge and procedure specific skills. Care must be provided in facilities which are fit for purpose and respect the privacy and dignity of patients. Each element of the clinic/patient interaction in a care pathway should be defined and described clearly in Standard Operating Procedures (see Section 14.4.4).

The *output* of the service will include some patients who will have become pregnant, and many who will not. All will have degrees of satisfaction in relation to their experience of the service. Analysis of the process of care at its various stages should identify areas of deficiency allowing corrective and preventative actions to be instituted enabling improved performance at all levels for the benefit of patients/users of services.

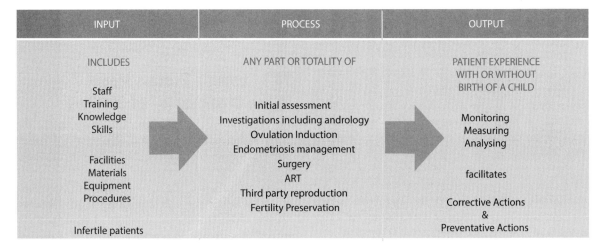

INPUT	PROCESS	OUTPUT
INCLUDES	ANY PART OR TOTALITY OF	PATIENT EXPERIENCE WITH OR WITHOUT BIRTH OF A CHILD
Staff Training Knowledge Skills	Initial assessment Investigations including andrology Ovulation Induction Endometriosis management Surgery ART Third party reproduction Fertility Preservation	Monitoring Measuring Analysing
Facilities Materials Equipment Procedures		facilitates
Infertile patients		Corrective Actions & Preventative Actions

Figure 14.1 Process mapping in fertility care.

14.4 Quality Management in Practice

The Quality Management System (QMS) should define the requirements of those seeking assistance, identify what the clinical service can offer, define and record the processes involved in the provision of the clinical service and establish quality objectives for the organisation. These will be aligned to the key issues of patient safety, clinical effectiveness, patient experience and regulatory compliance alluded to earlier.

The **quality policy** for the fertility service should clearly define the corporate and shared vision of those who work there. It should include the views and aspirations of all stakeholders. The quality policy might for example be a statement along the lines that

> This clinic aims to provide rational, efficient and effective treatment delivered in a compassionate manner to all our patients in accordance with UK regulatory requirements within an environment which is sensitive to the needs of patients and the staff who work within the Centre.

Managers in all areas of a clinical service should have input into the development of the Quality Policy. The QMS requires demonstration that standards related to the agreed Policy are met, for example, an aspiration to provide compassionate care will require supportive evidence of that being achieved most likely through patient feedback systematically researched through questionnaires.

There are a number of components which contribute to a quality management system within a fertility centre (Figure 14.2). Individually and collectively these ensure that services are provided in a consistent and effective way. These will be examined in detail.

14.4.1 Quality Objectives

The quality policy provides the framework upon which the clinic can build its quality objectives. These set out for the centre the principles upon which the quality policy aspirations will be realised. All should be patient focused and be inclusive of elements which support patients' emotional as well as physical needs in undertaking treatment. The acronym SMART is helpful in defining criteria in the setting of objectives. A **S**pecific area should be targeted for improvement. The objective should be **M**easurable to allow a determination as to whether progress is being made. Any aspirational target set should be **A**chievable and **R**ealistic, with improvement expected to occur within a defined **T**imeframe.

Examples of objectives which a clinic might set could include

- Improving live birth rates
  - This might be achieved through adjustments to clinical or laboratory protocols.
- Enhancing the patient experience
  - This might be achieved through a response to patient feedback on an element of care in a survey or by enhancing information provision.

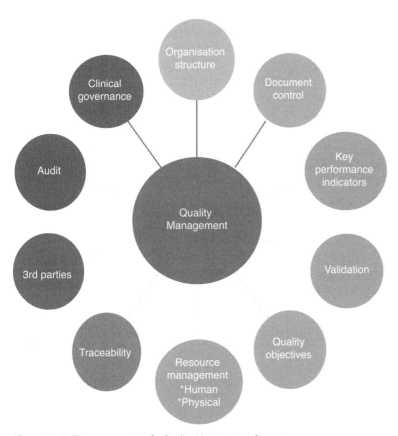

Figure 14.2 The components of a Quality Management System.

- Increasing the numbers of patients being seen
  - This might be achieved through adjustment to clinic schedules or referral pathways.
- Increasing staff satisfaction within the workplace
  - This might require adjustment to training policies, enhancing access to continuous professional development sessions, improving in-house communication pathways.

Setting objectives underpin a culture within a clinical service focused on improvement in performance.

14.4.2 The Quality Manager

Implementation of the QMS requires a sound organisational and management structure. A team of leaders in a fertility centre, whether administrative, clinical or laboratory based, are vital to the delivery of a quality-based service. While quality is a responsibility for all, appointment of an individual with lead responsibility for oversight of the QMS is essential. The Quality Manager (QM) is a key appointment within any organisation and is tasked to ensure that the QMS is functioning appropriately and effectively. This appointment is a regulatory requirement for treatment centres in the United Kingdom as dictated by the HFEA Code of Practice. Beyond that, it is also a regulatory requirement that laboratories undertaking diagnostic semen analysis should be certified to the ISO 15189:2012 standard, which also explicitly requires implementation of a QMS.

The QM should be an individual with effective communication skills and possessing high-level organisational skills. The QM should either be part of the management team or be able to report to management on how the QMS works and how effective it is. The QM needs to engage with all staff within the centre, encouraging co-operation with the principles of quality management and opening lines of communication both horizontally and vertically within and between all professional disciplines in the centre. The QM must institute and manage a robust document control system and ensure that the components of audit, performance review and continual improvement integral to the QMS are delivered. It is not expected that the QM carries out all these functions on their own but they, together with senior management, need to ensure that tasks in relation to these components are covered and delegated appropriately.

14.4.3 Organisational Structure

All components of the organisation involved in the process of care are accountable to the QMS. An organisational chart therefore needs to be all inclusive. Those contributing in clerical, administrative, medical, nursing, counselling, secretarial, domestic, andrology, embryology, marketing and finance roles must be included. Their individual and collective contribution to the process of care should be defined and where relevant performance against standards and protocols monitored. In addition, it is important that the organisational chart should define accountability and reporting relationships in the organisation. An example is shown in Figure 14.3. It should be emphasised that one size does not fit all. An individual centre providing services needs to analyse its reporting structures according to its own particular circumstances.

14.4.4 Document Control

The need for a good system of document control cannot be overemphasised. The document control system should be designed to control the approval, issue and distribution of new and revised documents as well as the removal of obsolete documents. The system will ensure there is quick access documents, whether electronically or physically, by relevant staff. Systems for archiving records should be in place in line with regulatory requirements for duration of storage. In some instances this can be for 30 years.

A comprehensive log of the documents relating to all spheres of activity within the day-to-day life of the fertility service needs to be maintained. An example of a document control system is shown in Figure 14.4. It includes a catalogue of all consent forms, laboratory sheets, guidelines (internal and external), forms, letters, patient information and Standard Operating Procedures.

Standard Operating Procedures (SOPs) set out the individual processes contributing to a mapped pathway of care of a patient undergoing treatment. It is essential therefore that all processes are identified and that those delivering the process contribute to its documentation and are aware of the existence of the SOP. In describing a process it is essential that all contributing procedures are identified which may involve members of staff from a variety of disciplines. A lead author must take responsibility for the preparation of the SOP which should be approved by a second member of staff. The document should have a clear scope and purpose, provide exact details of how a task is performed and be amenable to audit. It is important, and a condition of the licensing of clinics, that all documents within the centre are controlled. This means that only current versions should be available and systems should be in place to ensure obsolete versions are archived. When a specific SOP

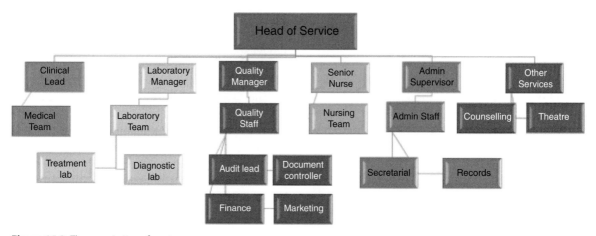

Figure 14.3 The organisation of services.

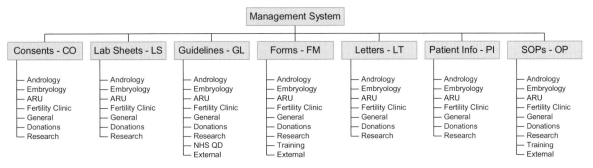

Figure 14.4 Document control within a Quality Management System.

needs to be updated it is the duty of the QM to ensure that the lead author is assigned to the task of review. Robust systems to reliably inform staff of any changes to an SOP need to be in place. Where required, team members provide input to the document and promote ownership of, and familiarity with, the SOP. Adherence to the components of the SOP is more likely in these circumstances.

Other key documents subject to control relate to Patient Information, Guidelines, Consent Forms, Laboratory Sheets, Correspondence and Forms. In the same way the QM needs to assign authorship to these documents such that review, usually on an annual basis, takes place. Each document is registered within the QMS and footers on the title page record its version number and date of creation, authorship, approval and planned review date.

Many hundreds of documents contribute to the QMS. Annual review of every document on an individual basis would be an enormous task and impractical. In the construction of a specific operating procedure a number of key documents associated with the procedure will be referenced within the text, for example, consent forms, patient information, correspondence, and so forth. These should be reviewed at the same time as the main SOP. Linked review thus streamlines the process.

Process maps also need to be created which detail how all protocols link to provide patients with cohesive treatment plans from the first encounter with the clinic to the conclusion of treatment. These key SOPs provide a link to all consent, lab sheets, guidelines, forms, letters and patient information.

14.4.5 Key Performance Indicators

Key performance indicators (KPIs) define the standards to which a clinical service aspires. They are based on measurable outcomes of activities undertaken within the service. Some, for example in the clinical and laboratory environment, will be informed by national guidelines which may have originated from professional bodies or the regulator. Others may be set by staff within the service. To ensure the whole team are engaged in working towards improving the quality of clinical care and outcomes, inclusive meetings should be held regularly to analyse KPIs relevant to clinical, laboratory and administration performance. There should be clear SOPs relating to which KPIs are in place for each area. A concern that a particular performance indicator is below an agreed standard should initiate a corrective action. Trends over time should also be explored and if a deterioration in performance is identified preventive action may be taken before a critical situation arises.

It is important therefore that the performance of the clinic as a whole as well as that of individuals be collected and regularly analysed. KPIs to assess should be agreed by senior management and will cover all areas within the organisation. Examples of areas for review could include

- Time from referral to appointment (administrative)
- % appointments missed at clinics (administrative)
- Average % motile sperm recovery in IUI treatment preparations (andrology)
- % initiated IVF cycles reaching egg recovery (clinical)
- % eggs fertilised with IVF or ICSI (embryology)
- % patients having egg recovery leading to cryopreservation (embryology)
- Embryo utilisation rate (embryology)
- Multiple pregnancies as % of all pregnancies (clinical)
- Cleaning schedules (domestic)

161

The list is by no means complete but each clinic will define for itself the specific KPIs which are integral to its needs. Guidance on appropriate KPIs is available from professional organisations such as the Association of Clinical Embryologists (ACE), the British Fertility Society (BFS) and the European Society for Human Reproduction and Embryology (ESHRE).

The generation of data, on its own, is not enough. Standards need to be agreed against which Quality Assurance processes can be initiated. Thus if a specific parameter falls below the agreed target an action pathway should be followed which sets in place an investigation as to possible contributing factors for the shortfall. If, for example, the number of eggs generated in stimulation cycles was below the expected level in a given period it would be legitimate to ask if this was because of patient characteristics, for example, age of the patient pool, the drug regime used to stimulate the ovaries, inexperience of the operator collecting eggs or any other factor? Remedial steps can then be put in place to address the issue and a further audit of performance can subsequently take place. These steps are the keys to *Quality Improvement* – setting standards, measuring performance, analysing performance, improving performance (Figure 14.5).

Monitoring the functioning of equipment in the laboratory is an important component of key performance monitoring. Data on the air quality and level of microbial contamination within the laboratory also need to be regularly collected. In addition, the other key components of pH and temperature regulation within the laboratory need to be monitored. It is particularly important to assess the impact of the introduction any changes in laboratory processes or equipment on these parameters.

14.4.6 Validation and Verification of Equipment and Processes

Whenever new equipment or materials are used in the clinic or laboratory it is essential that a rigorous validation process is followed. This includes reference to

- *User Requirements* (What do we need?)
- *Installation Qualifications* (Have we got what we need and does it work?)
- *Operational Qualifications* (What do we need to maximise utility?)
- *Performance Qualifications* (How do we check performance on an ongoing basis?)

An example might be the need for ultrasound scanning equipment. Is the proposed new scanning machine of an appropriate specification for the task required? When installed, is the scanner calibrated correctly? Are staff members trained and able to use it? Is the performance of the machine consistent and reliable and what maintenance schedule do we need?

In other words, it is an imperative to confirm through the provision of objective evidence that the requirements for a specific intended use or application have been fulfilled. In the United Kingdom, it is a requirement that all materials are CE marked where they are intended for in vitro processes.

This principle of checking before commissioning may be applied in a similar fashion to a process, to materials used in the laboratory or to the clinical/laboratory/environment in which care is provided.

14.4.7 Resource Management

14.4.7.1 Human Resources

Staff members are the most vital asset in any organisation and it is important that all personnel working in the centre feel valued and supported. To deliver effective care there must be a team approach within the fertility service as each discipline plays a part in the patient journey. Administrative, nursing, medical and laboratory staff must be aware of the relevance of their individual contributions to the overall performance of the service and the meeting of the quality objectives.

To achieve this all staff must have the skills required to meet their job description and where necessary

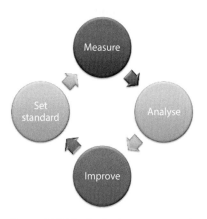

Figure 14.5 The Quality Improvement cycle.

develop skills as new techniques are introduced. Management have a responsibility to provide a supportive learning environment which encourages the professional development of all staff. Evidence should be documented when staff are appraised on an annual basis when their own personal development plans are made which includes training needs. Time to attend courses and access other essential learning resources should be provided. Personnel need to be competent to carry out the tasks assigned to them. There should be a documented procedure regarding the ratio of staff to service provision and what steps need to be taken should there be insufficient staff available.

14.4.7.2 Physical Resources

Premises should be catalogued in a floor plan which defines the scope of the building including the purpose of each room. This can be utilised as a fire plan. The environment in which care is given and staff members are employed needs to conform to regulatory standards. Adequate numbers of consulting rooms which afford patients privacy and dignity, and which are cleaned and maintained to a high standard are to be expected, that is, a cleaning schedule should be created in collaboration with relevant staff, completed daily and reviewed monthly. Storage of gametes and embryos needs to be secure in the laboratory. Conditions with respect to air quality should be monitored 24 hours per day, as should all key pieces of equipment in the laboratory such as incubators and storage tanks. These should be linked to an alarm system which calls out expert staff to deal with any unexpected and untoward changes in the environment. These systems should be externally reviewed on a regular basis as well as being subject to routine robust internal scrutiny. This would include daily data record and review to detect adverse trends at an early stage. The laboratory should be accessible only to staff that work in that area therefore security on all doors should be in place.

All equipment and technical devices need to be validated and regularly inspected according to manufacturers' instructions. Cleaning of equipment should be performed regularly and recorded within the QMS.

14.4.7.3 Traceability

It is a regulatory requirement that records are kept within the centre which permit the ability to trace the history, application or location of any material, that is, gametes/embryos. Thus there needs to be a documented process within the QMS to enable location, and identification of a cell during any step from procurement, through processing, testing and storage to distribution to a recipient or its disposal. This includes information on any products or material coming into contact with those cells during their journey through the pathway of care. Unique patient identification must be applied to all dishes, containers, and so forth used and all gametes and embryos stored should be clearly labelled. Any medication provided to a patient needs to be traceable to allow adequate investigation and an ability to ensure protection of others, for example, in the case of a drug-related adverse event.

14.4.7.4 Third-Party Agreements

Suppliers of services, materials and equipment used by the centre should be evaluated on an annual basis and contracts reviewed. It is essential that Third-Party Agreements are formalised and that suppliers confirm that their organisation is subject to a QMS-based approach to quality assurance.

14.4.8 Clinical Governance

Many factors can influence the success of a service. In the event of a concern with respect to clinical outcomes, detailed analysis of all factors potentially at play will be required. This will require reference to the process map of the particular pathway of care and is likely to involve staff across a variety of disciplines. This needs to be managed carefully and sensitively, bearing in mind the need to support staff in what can be a personally challenging situation.

A proportionate response to a concern with respect to performance may utilise a variety of strategies:

- Risk Management/Risk Assessment
- Audit
- Quality inspections undertaken by external organisations
- Quality sampling including feedback from users of the service
- Quality tours of work areas by senior management
- Review of Key Performance Indicators (see Section 14.4.5)
- External review and inter-centre/inter-laboratory comparisons

14.4.8.1 Risk Management/Risk Assessment

Risk management meetings should be arranged on a regular basis. These can play an important part in reducing hazards for users of the service. An incident of relevance to this process may include an event or circumstance that could have or did lead to unintended and/or unnecessary harm to a person and/or a complaint, or perhaps loss or damage to gametes or embryos. Clinical and non-clinical incidents will be included in Risk Management. During these meetings any incident reported will be investigated and compared to standard operating procedures or guidelines. Analysis of the incident will determine if there are issues relating to documentation, communication, staff deployment and training among others and whether specific actions need to be taken to prevent recurrence of the problem. Minutes of the meeting should be prepared, circulated within the centre and fed back to all team members. The actions required should be agreed by the management team and an implementation plan put in place. It is important that such investigations are conducted impartially and serve as an analysis of systems rather than be perceived as a trial of individuals.

Risk Assessment complements this process and is a method whereby the centre can identify and estimate the probability of significant hazards occurring for individuals or gametes/embryos. Through analysis of the potential degree of harm that might occur as a consequence of an untoward event and the probability of its occurrence it can be determined how the risk will be managed within the organisation. This will guide the clinic as to whether a defined risk on the basis of its degree of consequence (major to negligible) or likelihood of occurrence (rare to almost certain) can be accepted or needs to be acted upon.

14.4.8.2 Audit

Confirming that what the centre says it does, through SOPs and other documentation, is what it does in reality is clearly important. Audit, managed by the QM, is the method whereby senior management can ensure that actual performance adheres to documented procedures. It is a form of internal quality control and may relate to a specific procedure (internal audit) or a process. External audits such as that provided through the NEQAS system for andrology and embryology laboratories are additional resources.

Audits require to be planned and it would be expected that several would take place in each department within the organisation. It would be the responsibility of management within each section within a service to have an annual audit plan in place. A central register should be kept of all audits undertaken. Some audits may be unplanned or unannounced, and some may be provoked by circumstances such as an untoward incident or the adverse event affecting patient, gamete/embryo or staff safety. It is imperative that those carrying out the audit are trained for the task. They need to familiarise themselves with the documentation relating to the process being audited and observe the process being performed. Where deviations from the protocol are observed then these should be recorded. Typically a report will be written up by the auditors highlighting areas of non-conformance and comment made on potential corrective and preventative actions which can be taken. A time scale for the correction of non-conformity should be given and where required relevant SOPs should be re-written. Thereafter re-audit can be arranged if necessary, once more in line with the principle of facilitating continuous improvement. If a serious adverse event occurs such as a life-threatening complication associated with treatment a Root Cause Analysis exercise may be instituted. This involves detailed investigation involving input from all stakeholders and may shed light on avoidable factors leading to changes in clinical protocol, training of staff and adjustment to other components in the delivery of care.

14.4.8.3 Quality Inspections

In the United Kingdom, licensed Fertility Centres are inspected by HFEA on a regular basis. Some centres also have ISO 9001:2015 Quality Management Systems in place. Continued certification requires external surveillance assessment audits as part of a three-year plan. Centres providing diagnostic semen analysis services are now required to have ISO 15189:2012 certification and this also requires external audit.

14.4.8.4 Quality Sampling

This can be demonstrated by undertaking surveys of patient experience through questionnaires, feedback sessions as well as obtaining feedback from referring clinicians.

14.4.8.5 Quality Tours

These should be carried out on a regular basis by the QM and representatives of the management team.

These tours may include speaking to patients, staff, viewing facilities and meeting team leaders to review quality management engagement.

14.4.8.6 External Review

The HFEA publishes a report on an annual basis reviewing national data on outcomes of treatment. Data specific to all licensed centres within the United Kingdom are included. If a clinic perceives its performance as significantly at variance with national averages it may be useful to consider engaging with colleagues from other centres in an external review of the clinic. Such an exercise allows an independent view to be taken of the processes employed in the clinic, and advice on adjustments to protocols and procedures may be usefully given and received.

14.4.8.7 Data Protection

In the United Kingdom, the Data Protection Act 2018 came into force on 25 May 2018. General Data Protection Regulations now apply to all treatment centres which entail a statutory obligation to exercise care with patient data while being used or retained under the centre's control.

Information shared by users of the service is given in confidence. Documented procedures for identification, collection, indexing, access, storage, maintenance, amendment and safe disposal of records which contain patient identifying information need to be prepared. Stored data relating to patient treatment whether in hard copy or computer files must be secure and all staff should be aware of their legal responsibilities in this regard.

Centres will have in their possession information relating to donors and children born as a result of treatment. It is imperative that these data are kept confidential and disclosed only in the circumstances permitted by law. It is imperative that patients, their partners, and donors do not have access to any other person's records without first obtaining that person's consent.

14.5 Quality Review

At planned intervals senior managers within the organisation must review the QMS to determine whether it is adequate and effective. The review will cover the quality objectives which were set at the previous review and should include an assessment of the status of corrective and preventative actions

(CAPAs) previously agreed. These, together with the last period's KPIs, are discussed and where shortfalls in performance are identified determinations on new CAPAs are made.

In addition, a review of audits, risk management, external factors impacting on the centre's activities, training and education, as well as service delivery in several areas of the clinic and laboratory are discussed. The financial situation of the centre will be discussed and an analysis of present suppliers' performance made.

Action points for the following year are agreed upon and quality objectives set. This may include specific recommendations with respect to staff and equipment levels, audit activities to be arranged and provides clarity for everyone on the opportunities for improvement which exist. It is essential that feedback from the annual review is given to all members of the team. A feeling of shared ownership of these data is invaluable in maintaining a team ethos within a treatment centre.

14.6 Conclusion

Quality management systems became a statutory requirement for all UK IVF units only in the last 15 years. As such the imposition of what for many proved to be an expensive investment in terms of staff and IT infrastructure to support its introduction was a formidable challenge. The evidence underpinning the decision to demand this of IVF units in terms of improved success rates and greater numbers of babies was scant. The principles enshrined in QMS are widely practised in many areas of public service and it is generally accepted that clinics must strive for high and consistent standards of care as expected by increasingly well informed and articulate users of services. Most working in the sector believe that this is more likely to be achieved by keeping quality at the forefront of our approach to provision of healthcare. This should cover all the components in the service – all staff in all areas of centres providing infertility care. Measuring what we do, analysing performance and setting targets to improve should be fundamental to how we approach our work in contemporary clinical practice.

Further Reading

Alper MM. Experience with ISO quality control in assisted reproductive technology *Fertil Steril*. 2013;**100**:1503–8.

Dancet EAF, D'Hooghe TM, Spiessens C, Sermeus W, De NeuBourg D, Karel N, et al. Quality indicators for all dimensions of infertility care quality: consensus between professionals and patients *Hum Reprod.* 2013;**28**:1584–97.

ESHRE Special Interest Group of Embryology and Alpha Scientists in Reproductive Medicine. The Vienna consensus: report of an expert meeting on the development of art laboratory performance indicators. *Hum Reprod. Open.* 2017. DOI: 10.1093/hropen/hox011 1–17.

Human Fertilisation and Embryology Authority. *Code of Practice*, 9th ed. Revised January 2019. Available at: www .hfea.gov.uk/media/2793/2019–01-03-code-of-practice-9t h-edition-v2.pdf (accessed February 2019).

Human Fertilisation and Embryology Authority. Fertility Treatment 2014–2016 Trends and Figures. Available at: www.hfea.gov.uk/media/2563/hfea-fertility-trends-and-figures-2017-v2.pdf (accessed March 2019).

Olofsson JI, Banker MR, Sjoblom LP. Quality Management systems for your in vitro fertilization clinic's laboratory: why bother? *J Hum Rep Sci.* 2013;**6**:3–8.

World Health Organization. Quality of Care: A process for making strategic choices in health systems. Available at: www.who.int/management/quality/assurance/Quality Care_B.Def.pdf (accessed February 2019).

Index

167